HOW TO COPE
SUCCESSFULLY WITH

CROHN'S DISEASE

TOM SMITH

Wellhouse Publishing Ltd

First published in Great Britain in 2004 by
Wellhouse Publishing Ltd
31 Middle Bourne Lane
Lower Bourne
Farnham, Surrey GU10 3NH

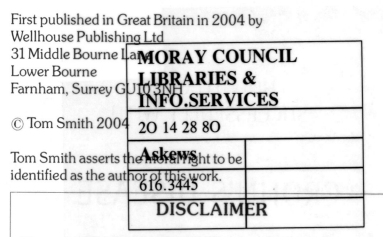

DISCLAIMER

The aim of this book is to provide general information only and
should not be treated as a substitute for the medical advice of
your doctor or any other health care professional. The publisher
and author is not responsible or liable for any diagnosis made by
a reader based on the contents of this book. Always consult your
doctor if you are in any way concerned about your health.

A catalogue record for this book is available from the British Library

ISBN 1 903784 16 6

Also by Dr Tom Smith in the How to Cope Successfully series:
  Colitis
  Depression
  Diabetes
  High Cholesterol
  Thyriod Problems

Printed and bound in Great Britain by
Creative Print & Design Group, Middlesex UB7 0LW

Contents

Preface 6

Introduction 7

1   The Normal Bowel – What it Does 9

2   Constipation 15

3   Diarrhoea 17

4   When the Diarrhoea Becomes Chronic –
    The Signs of Crohn's Disease and Colitis 30

5   Descriptions of Crohn's Disease 33

6   Crohn's – Why and How 41

7   Crohn's – Myths and Maybes 53

8   Eating with Inflammatory Bowel Disease –
    Tackling Food Intolerance 61

9   Ulcerative Colitis – A Background 67

10 Current and Future Treatments for Ulcerative Colitis 73

11 Ulcerative Colitis – The Need for Follow-up 77

12 Surgery for Colitis 81

13 Surgery for Crohn's Disease 85

14 Irritable Bowel and Coeliac Disease 89

    Appendix a Why You Mustn't Smoke –
    And How to Stop If You Do 97

    References 105

    Index 109

Dr Tom Smith

Having graduated from Birmingham Medical School, Dr Tom Smith spent two years in hospital house positions before entering general practice, first in Birmingham and then South Ayrshire. He then became medical adviser and later medical director of a major pharmaceutical company where he organized and helped to publish clinical trials of new drugs and took the Diploma in Pharmaceutical Medicine of the Royal College of Physicians of Edinburgh. Dr Smith has been a full-time writer since 1977 with many popular medical books to his credit (including Diabetes, High Cholesterol, Depression & Thyroid Problems for Wellhouse) together with weekly medical columns in several regional newspapers. He also finds time to practice as a locum for the family doctors in his home area of Girvan, Ayrshire, South West Scotland. Tom is married with two children.

Preface

When my publisher asked me to write two books, one on colitis and one on Crohn's disease, I at first demurred. One book covering both illnesses I felt was enough. They are similar illnesses, with similar symptoms and similar treatments, and I thought at first that people with one or other of these two common diseases would be interested in a single book that covered both.

I was persuaded to write two separate books by both my publisher and several patients. My publisher wanted two focussed books, clearly aiming at their readers. My patients most wanted to know about their own particular variety of bowel disease, and for me to focus on its causes and treatments.

So this is the second of my books on inflammatory bowel diseases – what used to be known graphically as the 'bloody fluxes', a name that today's sufferers would readily recognize as neatly describing their main symptoms. The first, *How To Cope Successfully with Colitis*, which deals mainly with ulcerative colitis, was published by Wellhouse Publishing in 2003.

Crohn's disease and ulcerative colitis are collectively known to doctors as 'inflammatory bowel disease', or IBD. Most lay people, however, would also link irritable bowel syndrome (not to be confused with IBD) and diverticular disease to colitis – and, of course, some people have the misfortune to have more than one of these conditions at the same time. In particular, irritable bowel and diverticular disease are a common combination. It is often difficult to persuade people with irritable bowel syndrome that this is all they have, that it is not true IBD, and that they do not have something more serious, such as cancer.

Most of this book is devoted to Crohn's, partly because there are already many books for people with irritable bowel, and few on IBD. But it would not be complete without chapters on how to distinguish IBD from irritable bowel, diverticular disease and colon cancer, the symptoms of all of which can mimic Crohn's. So it is aimed not just at Crohn's sufferers but also at people who have other conditions of the bowel and who may wish to know more about them.

Introduction

If you have repeated bouts of diarrhoea, with blood and mucus (like the nasal and throaty phlegm you get in the congestive stage of a cold) in it, then you probably have IBD. The two commonest causes of this combination of symptoms are Crohn's disease and ulcerative colitis. This book will concentrate on Crohn's disease, but it also has chapters on ulcerative colitis, mainly to explain their similarities and the differences between them. Its aim is to help you to understand what is happening in the course of IBD, and how modern medicine is used to relieve the symptoms and to prevent the serious complications that caused so many tragedies in the past.

To do this, the book starts by explaining how the normal bowel works. It shows how it can go wrong and how, if it becomes inflamed, it can produce the three main symptoms of diarrhoea, bleeding and mucus production. If they continue, your health deteriorates quickly: the book covers the methods by which doctors can correct them and help you towards recovery.

It also describes the tests and investigations you can expect in a modern gastroenterology unit, as your specialists first make the diagnosis and then estimate the extent of your illness. It is not just the illness that you have, but how much of your bowel is affected by it, that makes the difference to how you will be treated and how quickly and completely you will recover.

Other bowel problems that mimic Crohn's disease are described, so that you can relate your particular set of symptoms and test results to them. The section on irritable bowel is especially important, because many people with it are reluctant to accept their diagnosis without repeated tests that are bound to be negative. If you have been told you have irritable bowel and not Crohn's or colitis, please read the chapter on it and believe.

Finally, there is a section on the possible causes of Crohn's. It is as difficult for doctors as for their patients to accept that they do not yet know the causes of the diseases they are treating. The ideal is for us to establish the cause and treat it, so that the disease will be cured. We still do not know the causes of either Crohn's or ulcerative colitis, but we are getting closer to them. We do know, however, a lot about the changes that occur in the bowel of people with Crohn's, and how to return them to normal. It should be only a matter of time before we know why they happen, as well as what has happened.

Chapter One

The Normal Bowel – What it Does

First, a few definitions. The small intestine, or ileum, is the middle part of the gut, the whole of which is also known as the alimentary canal, the digestive tract or the gastroenterological system. That's why, when your general practitioner (GP) wants to investigate your bowel further, you will be referred first of all to a gastroenterologist. The ileum contains the liquidized remnants of your meals, which have already been semi-digested by the combined juices of the saliva, the stomach, the bile and the pancreas. In the ileum the process of digestion is completed, and all the nutrients – fatty acids (from fats in the food), amino-acids (from the food proteins) and glucose (from sugars and starches), as well as minerals and vitamins – are ready to be taken up through the ileum wall into the circulation. From there they pass to the liver, where they are turned into our own complex fats, proteins and glucose products.

By the time the contents of the ileum reach the end of the small intestine – the 'terminal ileum' (about which more later) – all the processes of digestion are completed. The residue then passes into the colon, where its water content is removed. By the time it reaches the lowest end of the colon, its contents are fully formed into the familiar solid stools that we normally pass once a day in normal health. Just how all this happens, and how the process can go wrong, needs to be explained before you can understand Crohn's disease.

The whole process of digestion of food, then expulsion of waste matter, is a dynamic one. First the food, then the remnants of digestion, are propelled onwards from mouth to anus by co-ordinated movements of muscles in the oesophagus (gullet), then the stomach, passing onwards to the small intestine (ileum), then the large bowel (colon) and then to the rectum and anus. The co-ordination is controlled by messages from nerves inside the gut walls and by chemical 'messengers' secreted into the bloodstream by cells in the lining layers of the stomach and small bowel, in response to the appearance of food higher up. Sensitive tissues in the wall of the colon detect these messengers in the blood, and react to them by causing its muscles to contract. This pushes onwards the material inside it.

To start at the beginning: we take food or drink into our mouths, and with a conscious act, we use the muscles in our throat to swallow it. From that moment onwards, we are relatively unconscious, apart from noticing an occasional gurgle, of the food's progress through our gut – until we feel the need to expel it from the rectum and anus perhaps a day later. Yet the gut is doing a lot of work to make sure we get the maximum benefit from what we have eaten.

You probably think that once we swallow something, it slips down into the stomach by gravity. Not so. As students we had a tutor who disproved this neatly by standing on his head and drinking a pint of beer upside down. He probably enjoyed the lecture more than we did. He didn't mind doing an encore. It's unlikely that he would be allowed to make such a demonstration today. Sadly most medical students now learn from video presentations rather than from real live lecturers.

His point was that food and drink moves from the back of the mouth into the stomach by a ripple, like a wave, of muscular contractions of the oesophagus – the tube inside the chest that connects the throat to the stomach. These contractions push the food onwards regardless of the position of the person doing the swallowing. They certainly work in space, too, with no gravity. Astronauts have no trouble swallowing and digesting food.

From the oesophagus, the food enters the stomach, just under the diaphragm. The stomach is a very active organ, churning and mixing the food so that its surface comes into contact with every portion of it. In the stomach's surface are cells that secrete acid and other digestive juices that are poured over the food to start the process of digestion. The crucial part of this process is that the stomach only becomes active when it receives the appropriate messages to do so. This is where the principle that guides the whole digestive system in normal health comes in. That is, that what is happening higher up in the gut produces signals to the next part of the gut, lower down, to be ready for action.

For most of the day and night, the stomach is relatively inactive. Its muscles are relaxed, its secretory cells are producing very little digestive juice or acid, and there are only a few odd 'ripples'. But start to eat, or even begin to salivate at the thought of the next tasty meal, and chemical messengers are released from the mouth into the bloodstream to stir the stomach into action.

To put it simply, food in the mouth starts the stomach working. Food hitting the stomach 'kick starts' all the processes in the ileum, and in organs like the gallbladder and pancreas, that will complete the process of digestion. The same process, food reaching the stomach, sends off messages to the large bowel – the colon – to push its contents forwards to the rectum and anus, so that the stool can be expelled. This is called the gastro-colic reflex. Its purpose is simple: with more food in the stomach to be digested, the colon needs to be emptied to make room for it.

For most of the day, the rectum is usually empty. When we wake in the morning and eat breakfast, the chemical message from stomach to the left half of the colon causes it to push any material inside it into the rectum. We feel that pressure inside the rectum, and have the desire to empty it. So we sit down – in the process straightening out the angle between the rectum and the anus. The faeces can then enter the anus, and are expelled by our conscious use of the stomach-wall muscles and internal muscles called the levatores ani. This not only empties the anus, but also means that all the faeces stored in the left half of the colon will be passed, too.

Most of us in health pass around 150 to 300 millilitres of faeces each day. However, if we decide to refuse to obey the bowel's message that it wants to be emptied (sometimes the message comes at an awkward time), the rectum can expand to accommodate as much as 400 millilitres. It may even go 'into reverse' for a while, so that the faeces are driven back and upwards into the sigmoid colon. If we make a habit of doing this, the result is chronic constipation. It is best, if we can, to accede to our colon's first request.

The colon

The colon is 1.5 metres (nearly 5 feet) long. It is a closed tube. The small bowel, or ileum, empties into it through a valve (the 'ileo-caecal valve') so that once the food residue has passed from the small to the large bowel, it cannot pass backwards again.

It has four distinct parts. The first is the ascending colon, that passes upwards from the lower right quarter of the abdomen to the area under the lower right ribs. It then turns a right angle to become the transverse colon, that runs from right to left across the upper abdomen. At the end of this second part of the colon it turns downwards, through another right angle, to become the descending colon, running down the left half of the abdomen. The final part of the colon is the 'sigmoid' (so named because of its resemblance to the Greek letter sigma – the equivalent to our letter 's'), which lies in the pelvis and leads to the rectum and anus. Where the sigmoid colon

The Digestive System

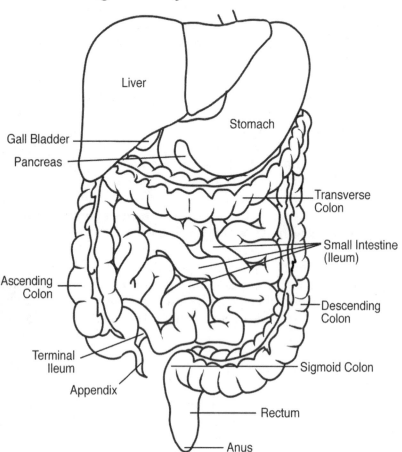

becomes the rectum there is another 'valve', or to be more accurate a 'sphincter', which holds the rectum and colon in place within the pelvis and contains some of the muscles we use in defecation. At this point, for the first time since we had the food in our mouth, we become conscious of, and have control over, the contents of our gut.

The rectum then leads to the anus, the last 5 centimetres in men and 4 centimetres in women, of the gut. The distinction between rectum and anus is very important for people with colitis, because the rectum is lined with glandular tissues, in contrast to the skin-like lining of the anus. As colitis is mainly a disease of glandular tissues, this explains why the rectum can be affected but the anus spared. Recently this knowledge has led to new surgical approaches to diseases like ulcerative colitis.

Throughout its length, the colon is supplied with blood vessels and nerves that control and co-ordinate the work of the muscles and glands in its wall. In normal health, the colon dehydrates (removes water from) the liquid end-products of digestion that it receives from the small intestine or ileum. To do this it needs to have a normal layer of lining cells. These cells, collectively called the epithelium, work selectively to take back into the body large amounts of water, salts and minerals, while allowing the waste products to be concentrated into what we all know as a normal motion, or 'stool'. Muscle contractions in the colon wall push the drying motion onwards towards the rectum and anus.

The muscle contractions are co-ordinated by 'plexuses' or networks of nerves within the colonic walls. Electrical impulses generated by these plexuses cause the muscles from the ascending to the sigmoid colon to contract in sequence, so that the shift is almost always towards the rectum, from which the final fully formed stool can be expelled.

Chapter Two

Constipation

In animals and in primitive humans – our ancestral hunter-gatherers of only a few thousand years ago – the call to empty the bowel was naturally followed by a moment's stop to do just that. We deposited a stool something like a cow pat, and then we walked on. Our progress towards civilized living was the first step to abnormal bowel function. It became much more convenient to devote a particular time of day to a once-daily bowel evacuation. That meant training the body to ignore the 'call' after each meal. Most people settle for a motion just after breakfast. Because the faeces of modern humans remain longer inside the colon, they have became more dehydrated, and therefore less fluid. The cow pat was replaced by the sausage-like stool that most of us pass today.

Constipation

A once-a-day stool has become the norm, although it isn't necessarily 'normal' in the sense that it is physiologically correct. It means retaining the faeces inside the left half of the colon for up to 24 hours at a time. That's fine most of the time, but people who ignore their need to empty their bowel for much longer than that can get into the habit of chronic constipation. The longer the faeces remain inside the colon, the drier, and therefore harder, they become. And that can mean it is more difficult and uncomfortable to pass them when you do decide to open your bowel.

The Victorians saw this as unhealthy, which is why so many of their medicines were laxatives. Today we don't see constipation as a threat to health, but we aren't happy about regular laxative consumption. Most laxatives work by causing the bowel-wall muscles to contract, so that they may even go into spasm or cramp, giving rise to colic. That's why many laxatives cause stomach pains, and people even judge them by the cramp they feel when they have 'a good clean out'. The older generation who grew up with daily laxatives being fed to them by their well-meaning but quite mistaken parents may still feel a laxative isn't any good unless it causes a bit of stomach ache in the process.

In fact, the bowel gets used to daily laxatives, so that it eventually stops responding to the normal signals of a full rectum. A vicious circle starts, in which higher and higher doses of laxatives are taken: the end result is a flaccid bowel which is very difficult to empty. The only recourse is to stop the laxatives and try to re-educate the person into a more normal bowel habit.

Why do I bring this information here, in a book on Crohn's disease? Because the information we have gathered from the huge numbers of people with constipation over more than a hundred years has clearly refuted the most common misconception about the cause of bowel disease. That is that so-called 'toxins' in the bowel, from germs in the contents of the gut, whether in the small or large bowel, are responsible for the inflammation that makes people so ill with ulcerative colitis or Crohn's disease.

In constipation, the germs inside the faeces are in much longer contact with the bowel wall, and are present in far greater numbers, than in people who have a regular once-daily motion. If germ-produced toxins were responsible for bowel disease, then people with constipation should surely have a far higher risk of developing it. Yet they don't. All that constipation causes is discomfort – it is not a cause of ill health. All that expense laid out by the famous (two royal ladies were apparently recent devotees) on regular colonic irrigation is for nothing. There is no need to irrigate the normal bowel: it is very capable of evacuating itself, very efficiently.

ChapterThree

Diarrhoea

This is where explaining bowel function in lay language becomes difficult. Having read so far, you could be forgiven for thinking that diarrhoea is just the opposite of constipation. In people with diarrhoea, you might think, the material that the colon collects from the small intestine has simply reached the rectum too quickly to be dehydrated enough, so you pass a loose stool. You would then follow up that logic with the conclusion that the colon is over-active, pushing its contents onwards too fast.

Sadly, the mechanism of diarrhoea isn't as simple as that, particularly not in colitis. In fact, in many people with colitis the colon is almost inactive, with a flabby, almost inert muscular activity. There are complex changes in the colitic bowel that need to be explained if you are to understand your own condition and help yourself to combat it. So please don't skim over this section: it is important to understand it.

First, we have to define diarrhoea. That's not as easy as it seems. For example, most of us would agree that it is opening the bowels more often than normal. But what is normal? For the hunter-gatherer mentioned above, it could be several soft stools a day. For most modern adults normality is a stool once a day, usually after breakfast. Yet there are many who pass stools healthily twice a day or once every two days.

So diarrhoea relates to your own previous experience: if you are passing stools much more often than you are used to, you may be developing diarrhoea. However, if the stool is fully formed, and not runny, that may not be a true diarrhoea. The motion must also be looser – more watery – than before. The watery component is quite important. Some people with irritable bowel, for example, describe what they pass as 'diarrhoea' when it is really a stream of tiny firm pellets, similar to rabbit droppings. This is not diarrhoea, and could even be interpreted as a form of constipation!

For the purposes of this book, therefore, diarrhoea can be taken to mean both passing stools more often than is usual for you and that the stools are more watery than usual. We have all had it. Most of us at some time have had gastroenteritis – a bout of sickness and diarrhoea that has followed some dietary indiscretion. There are dozens of circumstances by which people can develop gastroenteritis. Eating undercooked thawed-out frozen meat, particularly poultry or shellfish, is a common cause. Kitchen staff who are not fastidious enough about their hygiene are another.

Common to all these dining disasters is a germ that has either been inside the raw food, or has been smeared on it by dirty kitchen utensils or unwashed hands. If the process of cooking isn't complete, some of the germs are encouraged to multiply in the warmth, and they can then infect your gut in such numbers they make you ill.

But why is the illness diarrhoea? That's what this book is all about, because an understanding of the processes that lead to diarrhoea is crucial to your understanding of your colitis. They all depend on the integrity – the good health – of the cells that form the inner lining of the gut. The name of these cells as a tissue is the epithelium, and the cells themselves are mucosal cells – so called because they secrete mucus, the slimy liquid in which the digestive processes take place. Another word for the epithelium is the mucosa.

The mucosa, from the stomach to the anus, is a very active organ in its own right. It is the regulator of how much fluid we pass, eventually, in our stools. To understand why it is so crucial, we need to know something of how it controls our fluid balance. So let's take a journey from mouth to anus, measuring the flow of water as we do so. The food we chew and send down to our stomachs is a semi-solid mass. The stomach adds a lot of acid juices, so that by the time it reaches the duodenum, the first part of the gut past the stomach, it is much more fluid, probably more than double the volume of the food you have swallowed. You pass around 7 to 8 litres (15 pints) of fluid from your stomach into the duodenum in a normal day.

If you think this is a lot of fluid, then consider that to this volume is added juices entering the duodenum from the bile ducts (from the liver and gallbladder) to start the digestion of fats, and from the pancreas to continue the digestion of proteins and sugars. At the same time the mucosal cells of the small intestine are pouring their mucus and watery juices into the cavity within the bowel. Doctors call this cavity, in which the fluid flows, the lumen. The volume of the

Microscopic appearance of slice through normal intestine

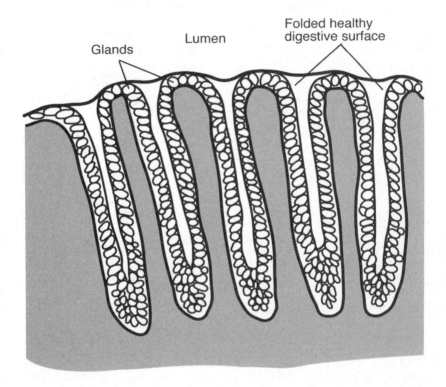

Glands

Lumen

Folded healthy digestive surface

material in your bowel lumen, by the time it gets to the end of the small intestine and is ready to enter the colon through the ileo-caecal valve, is around 10 to 15 litres a day.

However, this isn't just a passive flow of fluid from the mucosa into the small bowel. The mucosal cells are working hard, pumping exactly the correct concentrations of minerals (the technical term is electrolytes), such as sodium, potassium and chloride, across their outer membranes – the surfaces that face the lumen in which are the bowel contents.

In good health, the mucosal cells make sure that we get the balance of sodium and potassium, and water, in our bloodstream exactly right, within a very small margin. Recently we have discovered that zinc is also vital – but more about that later. To keep this balance so

Microscopic appearance of slice through area of colitis/ Crohn's
(note loss of glands and digestive surface)

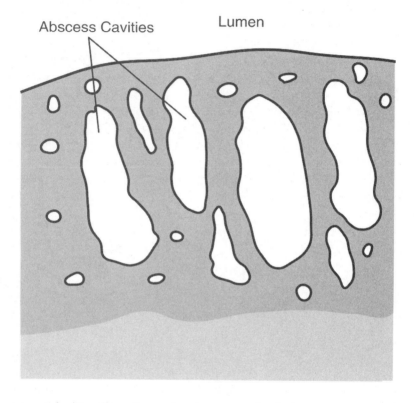

accurately, literally gallons of water pass in both directions across the mucosa, between your circulation and the contents of your bowel, every day.

You can see, with an electron microscope, the tiny gaps in the mucosal cell surface membranes (in effect their walls) through which the electrolytes are pumped, along with the water in which they are dissolved. The chemical substances, or enzymes, produced either by the body itself in the normal process of digestion or by invasive germs in infections, which 'open' and 'shut' these gaps, can be examined in detail. The technical details of how this can be done are well outside the remit of this book, but you can be assured that virtually everything is now known about how mucosal cells control the substances that pass through them, and what happens to them when things go wrong.

A good example of that knowledge and how we have put it to excellent use is the modern treatment of cholera. Today we in the developed world look on cholera as a rather exotic tropical disease, vaccination for which is one of the nuisances we must put up with when we are going on a tropical holiday. We couldn't be more wrong. In the middle of the nineteenth century it was rife throughout Britain. People with cholera died from terrible diarrhoea until the public health authorities closed down all the sources of contaminated water and piped clean water to all our cities.

However, cholera is certainly not a disease of the past. It still affects millions of people around tropical and subtropical areas of the world where the water supply is poor and people find it difficult, if not impossible, to follow all the good hygiene rules. I don't want to dwell on how people get infected with germs that cause diarrhoea, as this isn't what the book is about. However, what the cholera germ does to the mucosa of the ileum isn't too far from what happens in Crohn's disease, and may help you to understand what is going on when you have an acute attack, and why you get such severe diarrhoea.

Cholera is spread by a bacterium which is called a Vibrio, because it has a curly 'tail' when seen under a microscope that vibrates to propel the germ forwards. Vibrios secrete from their surface a substance that could be called an 'anti-enzyme' that 'blocks' – in other words switches off – the mucosal cells' ability to suck water and electrolytes back through the bowel wall from the lumen into the bloodstream. So the normal two-way flow of water across the bowel wall becomes entirely one-way – from body fluids into the lumen.

If you consider that this flow can be around 20 to 30 litres in a day, you can see that the Vibrio can create a tidal wave of fluid that has to be expelled as a mass of watery faeces. In a few hours, if that fluid is not replaced, the cholera victim simply dries up – he or she becomes like a withered plant in dire need of extra water and electrolytes. Until we began to understand this process, cholera killed people simply by dehydrating them. Even when we gave antibiotics to kill off the cholera germ, it could take too long for the mucosal cells to recover, and its victims still died. Now we know better. Instead of dosing patients with antibiotics, in very severe cases we replace all the lost fluid very quickly by giving drips into the patients' veins. We let the body's own immune defences tackle theVibrio, and as long as we can keep the patient in good water and electrolyte balance we can virtually guarantee a cure.

Cholera is the worst of the diarrhoeal infections because its attack on the mucosa is so overwhelming. But the fact that even it can be controlled by rehydration – replacing the water and electrolytes lost in the diarrhoea – has established such fluid replacement as the main objective of all diarrhoeal illnesses. If we can keep the whole body's fluid balance correct, and take the stress off the bowel, it will usually heal itself. So when family doctors in Britain are faced with patients with the usual, much less severe, forms of diarrhoea due to gastroenteritis, they normally give plenty of watery fluids along with the correct concentrations of glucose and electrolytes.

If you have had travellers' diarrhoea in recent years, you will surely recognize trade names such as *Rehydrat*, *Electrolade* and *Dioralyte* – all powders that when dissolved in a cup of water provide just what is needed. The mucosa doesn't have to expend any energy to 'digest' them, and the cells can recover quickly. Meanwhile, the diarrhoea can continue until all the infecting germs are expelled. Once they have gone, the mucosa soon returns to normal and the diarrhoea stops.

Today we hardly ever prescribe antibiotics or anti-diarrhoeal drugs for this form of diarrhoea. The antibiotics may lead to bacterial resistance, and anti-diarrhoeal drugs may only prolong the infection. They may ease the diarrhoea but make you feel a lot worse.

There are exceptions: for instance, typhoid fever which is caused by a germ called *Salmonella typhi*. The cholera germ stays within the lumen and the gut mucosal cells. It doesn't stray beyond these limits. That's why we can safely allow it to run its course. But salmonella doesn't stick to these limitations. While it initially causes severe diarrhoea and fever in the acute phase of the illness, it may also spread further, beyond the gut, into the bloodstream, and from there on into the gallbladder and kidneys. Once into the bloodstream it can cause overwhelming infection: the germs secrete poisons, or 'toxins', that can cause death in the acute phase. Prince Albert was one of its victims.

However, survivors of the initial typhoid infection may not get off lightly. The bacteria survive quietly, causing no problems, in the kidneys and gallbladder. Years after the original infection has settled and the person is apparently cured, living salmonella bacteria can still be shed from the gallbladder into the faeces and from the kidneys into the urine. These excretions are highly infectious, yet the person passing them feels perfectly well.

This is the salmonella 'carrier state'. Salmonella carriers have been for hundreds of years the instigators of typhoid outbreaks throughout the world. The most famous was 'Typhoid Mary' who lived in the United States in the nineteenth century. Unfortunately she tended to take work in kitchens, and moved on whenever an outbreak appeared around her. The story goes that she was identified and refused to stay away from food preparation: she did not believe that she could be responsible. Chased from state to state by the authorities, it is rumoured that she was eventually 'done away with'. She certainly disappeared from society in a mysterious way.

Typhoid fever is only one member of a family of salmonella infections. Others include *Salmonella paratyphi*, which causes paratyphoid fevers that can be just as lethal, and *Salmonella typhimurium*, or mouse typhoid, which can also attack humans. All can turn their victims into carriers, so it is usual to treat them with the correct antibiotics that kill not only the germs in the gut but also those that have lodged in the other organs. The drug of first choice nowadays is ciprofloxacin, but much depends on the laboratory tests on cultures of the germs, about which more later.

Salmonella was made famous throughout Britain, of course, when Edwina Currie, then a member of the government, claimed that most eggs and battery hens were infected with it. For telling what turned out later to be the truth, she lost her job and her future as a politician. It is still true that a substantial number of salmonella infections are caught from eating poultry, either contaminated during slaughter or as it is being prepared in the kitchen, or because the birds have been fed salmonella-infected feed. Outbreaks of salmonella have been traced to infected fishmeal from Peru, contaminated cocoa beans from West Africa (you don't want to know what was put on the fields as fertilizer), and seagull droppings on reservoirs after the gulls have been visiting sewage works and landfill sites.

Salmonella has a cousin that is much less well known to the general public. This is shigella. Shigella is the cause of bacterial dysentery – dysentery being the medical word for extremely severe diarrhoea. It was named after the Japanese doctor, Dr Shiga, who in the 1890s first described it as a cause of an epidemic of illness in which a quarter of its victims died. Shigella shuns other animals: it is only found in the gut of apes, monkeys and man. And as few of us have close contact with our fellow primates, the only way we can catch it is to eat food that has been contaminated by someone who has been less than hygienic.

That isn't as easy as it sounds. When we eat a chicken contaminated with salmonella, it is usually teeming with the germs. They need to be present in their thousands for them to cause an illness. There are several reasons for this. One is that the stomach is a pretty hostile environment for bacteria. It is extremely acid, so that bacteria that can't tolerate acid too well die very quickly. The stomach juices also contain the very powerful protein-digesting juice pepsin. The germs have to be protected against that, too, or they will become just part of the food chain. After all, they are made of protein.

So when salmonella invade us, they have to be present in reasonably large numbers, because only a small proportion of them survive the passage through the stomach. The ones that do make it through are probably protected by being thoroughly mixed with milk or masticated meat, so that they are not exposed to the destructive juices. It isn't so for shigella. Shigella bacteria have a considerable advantage over salmonella. They don't mind the acid environment. They survive the potential attack by pepsin, so you only need to swallow a few of them to develop a severe infection. A little lack of cleanliness after using the toilet, and your hands may have on their surface enough shigella germs to make the clientele of a whole restaurant sick. When you hear of a cruise liner with a diarrhoea epidemic, or a plane in which half the passengers were ill, shigella germs are high on the list of suspected infecting organisms. That brilliant scene in the spoof disaster movie *Airplane* in which all the pilots fell sick was pretty close to the mark.

Shigella comes in two forms – *dysenteriae* and *sonnei*. The first was the one described by Dr Shiga: the second was discovered later, and is less severe. But both cause fierce and very unpleasant diarrhoea that often needs emergency treatment, and that can lead to a form of true, lasting colitis. After a few days of watery diarrhoea and vomiting, the symptoms of shigella infection change. The vomiting stops, and you start to have bouts of colic. These are sudden cramps, deep inside the abdomen and rectum, that you find easiest to relieve by passing, many times a day, a small motion that is less watery, but streaked with blood.

This is a sign that the germ has passed from the small bowel to the colon, where it has started to infect the mucosal cells. The bleeding comes from many small ulcers – patches of raw mucosa that have been stripped of their lining, epithelial cells by the infection. In effect, the shigella infection has caused an acute colitis virtually identical to the condition seen in ulcerative colitis, about which you will read much more later.

Then there is E. coli. The E stands for Escherichia, after Dr Escherich, the German doctor who discovered it. When I was learning bacteriology as a medical student, E. coli was accepted as a normal constituent of the colon of humans and cows. It is only in recent years that we have recognized that some strains of it are far from benign. People have died from it in outbreaks of food poisoning, in which the beef responsible was contaminated at the abattoir – by careless removal of the animal's internal organs. The worst of these outbreaks was in the 1990s, in Wishaw, Scotland, where the outbreak was traced to contaminated beef, in which the same cutting utensils had been used for raw and cooked meats.

The lethal form of E. coli has a different approach to infection from those of cholera and typhoid. It doesn't travel beyond the gut wall, but it has two unpleasant properties. The first is that it has found a way to stick to the surface of the mucosal cells. That protects it from being washed away in the diarrhoea it causes. The second is that, once stuck to the cells it produces toxins to destroy the cells, so that it can use the residues of the dead cells, as nutrient on which it can thrive and multiply. Once the E. coli bacteria have started to multiply, they quickly spread throughout the bowel, stripping more mucosa from it. The toxins can now pass easily through the areas of denuded lining into the bloodstream, from where they cause serious damage to the kidneys, brain and other organs.

A less common, but particularly important, diarrhoea-causing bacterium is Yersinia enterolytica. Its importance lies in the fact that it seems to restrict itself to infecting a short area of small intestine just above the ileo-caecal valve, giving rise to a condition known as terminal ileitis. The 'terminal' here refers to the final part of the ileum, and not to the fact that the illness might be terminal! As Crohn's disease usually starts at precisely this part of the gut, and may even be limited to it, a Yersinia infection can easily be mistaken for Crohn's disease. That is a serious mistake, because Yersinia (but not Crohn's) is curable with the appropriate antibiotic. It is vital, when dealing with a bloody diarrhoea, not to miss an easily treatable condition.

So far, all the germs mentioned here have been bacteria. They are only part of this complex story. We haven't started yet on the other infections that cause diarrhoea – protozoa and viruses. Protozoa are single-celled parasites, prototype animals, that infect other animals by getting into their tissues. Probably the best known of them is the malaria parasite, plasmodium, which in its various forms causes the four main types of malaria. Plasmodia are injected under the skin by mosquito bites and target the red blood cells, and their life-cycle within us from then on causes the disease that has killed more human beings than any other illness.

Less well publicized are the amoebae, similar single-cell organisms that inhabit water. Generations of biology students in British schools have studied pools of pond-water and been fascinated by the free-living amoebae they can see under the high-power lenses of their microscopes. Those amoebae are usually benign, but they have much less benign relatives that we call entamoebae histolytica. They, like shigella, can manage to pass unscathed through the acid stomach environment.

'Ento' refers to the fact that these amoebae flourish inside an animal's (i.e. our) gut. The prefix 'histo' refers to cells (histology is the microscopic study of cells), and 'lysis' is the dissolving away of cells. So from the name it is fairly easy to deduce that the main property of entamoeba histolytica is its ability to dissolve away the human cells with which it comes into contact. In our gut, these are our mucosa cells. So the first achievement of an entamoeba infection is to remove from the gut lining an area of mucosa – causing an ulcer.

This isn't all. Once safely ensconced in the small bowel wall, the entamoeba uses the nutrient it gets from our dying cells first to multiply like fury, then to create a protective skin around the 'daughter' cells, preventing us from digesting them. They can then safely travel further down the gut to the colon, where they create havoc. The whole surface of the colon becomes infected and ulcerated, producing a bloody diarrhoea and making the unfortunate victim very ill. This is amoebic dysentery, and is still a major cause of death in countries where the water supply is not clean or the basic rules of hygiene are not kept.

Another protozoon, giardia lamblia, is a particular favourite of medical students. With a heart-shaped body and a few wispy 'hairs' projecting from its rear, it looks under the microscope just like a tiny face. It's not so funny if you swallow it in your drinking water, however. It has a predilection for the upper part of the small intestine, from where it can cause a very troublesome and sometimes bloody diarrhoea. It used to be confined mainly to Scandinavia and to the countries of the old Soviet Union, but in recent years it has spread as people have travelled. The main source used to be raw fish, a delicacy in some northern countries that is probably best avoided unless you can be sure that the fish is parasite-free. Marination may not kill parasites in fish flesh: adequate cooking always does.

As for viruses, not a year passes without researchers discovering yet another virus infection that causes diarrhoea. Viruses, of course, are much smaller than bacteria, and are not seen with conventional light microscopes. They need to be inside a living host cell to survive and multiply. Only a generation ago, when I and my contemporaries were training as doctors, viruses weren't thought to be a cause of diarrhoea. We knew they caused colds: in fact we knew of dozens of families of viruses that caused colds. We knew that viruses caused diseases like smallpox, chickenpox, herpes, hepatitis and types of meningitis. But we shunned the diagnosis of 'gastric flu', because we thought that viruses didn't go in for gut infections.

We couldn't have been more wrong. Around 1973 we learned about rotaviruses. They turned out to be the commonest cause of outbreaks of diarrhoea in babies' wards and nurseries in hospitals. Adults are less susceptible to rotavirus infections, probably because we become immune to infections with them in childhood. So rotaviruses are not seen as an important cause of acute colitis in adults. However, they were a pointer to the fact that there might be many more viruses that could inflame the gut – and so it proved. Winter epidemics of gastric flu may well be just that – a flu-like virus infection that is transferred not by swallowing contaminated food but by being breathed in from coughs and sneezes.

Although we don't yet know the details of all the viruses that can cause diarrhoea, we do know what happens to the bowel when they

27

attack. Bowel mucosa biopsies taken from patients during outbreaks show that the mucosal cells are abnormal. They have stopped producing their digestive enzymes and mucus. The result is that most of the sugar and fats in the food, plus a whole lot of water, remains to be passed on into the colon. The 'osmotic' pressure that the food residue of fatty acids and glucose exerts in the lumen sucks even more fluid from the circulation. The colon cannot perform its main function of dehydrating its contents, and the inevitable result is diarrhoea.

Where the viruses lodge in the intestine is difficult to pinpoint, but they are probably hidden within the mucosa of the first few feet of the small intestine, the upper part of the ileum. What we do know about viruses in general is that they do their damage by entering the cells themselves and multiplying there, after which they spread to infect the neighbouring cells. They do not produce a long-lasting toxin. Once your body's immune system has got rid of them, the diarrhoea stops.

Virus gastroenteritis is probably the cause of many cases of travellers' diarrhoea. If you have had it on holiday you will know from bitter experience that it can lay you flat for two or three days. Your only wish is to be near a toilet, and to have as much water as you can to drink, to replenish the fluid that you have lost. The best way to manage it is to keep drinking safe water and to add to it the glucose and minerals mentioned above several times a day.

Here is where we mention cruise ships again. The *Lancet*[1] reported on an investigation into gastroenteritis on cruise ships. The good news is that diarrhoea outbreaks on cruise ships have fallen from 27 per 100,000 passengers in 1975-79 to 3.5 per 100,000 in 1996-2000. This is partly because crew are much better trained and overseen in their handling of food and personal hygiene, and because the cruise lines are very much aware of the need for the highest standards of sanitation.

Even so, some viruses slip through the net because they are spread not through food, but by droplet infection. So no matter how fastidious the crew and passengers are, if someone brings an infection on board, it will spread like wildfire in the confined atmosphere of a crowded ship. The whole world heard about the *Aurora* in the summer of 2003 and the refusal of the Greek authorities to allow the passengers to land in Athens. In that outbreak around 400 of the 1,800 passengers went down with diarrhoea. Like the other episodes reported in recent years, aboard the *Amsterdam*, *Disney Magic*, *Carnival Fascination* and *Oceana*, the infection was due to viruses related to the 'Norwalk' virus, which also stalks hospitals in wintertime throughout the United Kingdom. Once the virus is on the ship, some crew members can become symptomless carriers, and spread it to future passengers.

The *Lancet* adds that the International Council of Cruise Lines is extremely aware of the problem. Spokeswoman for the Council Christine Fischer says that in the cruise industry every case is reported. The companies are doing all they can to reduce the figures further, with measures such as asking the crew to wash their hands at least every two hours. Sadly, to eliminate all the risk of a virus-induced diarrhoea, they would have to ask the crew not to breathe, too – hardly a practical step.

Antibiotics are not recommended for acute diarrhoea unless the condition continues past the first two days or becomes serious and there is a suspicion of salmonella or similar severe infection. Nor are there antibiotics that you can take to prevent an infection. Antibiotics do not work against viruses, and as mentioned above, if the cause is bacterial, you may just induce resistance, and become a carrier, if you take the wrong dose or the wrong antibiotic. If you have a lot of colicky pain with the diarrhoea, there is a case for taking drugs that will ease the spasm in the gut. The two most usual are diphenoxylate and loperamide. Many people take antibiotics or an anti-spasm drug routinely on holiday on the assumption that it will prevent travellers' diarrhoea. Neither will do that: there is no case for taking preventive medicines.

Chapter Four

When the Diarrhoea Becomes Chronic – The Signs of Crohn's Disease and Colitis

Having read so far, you will probably have recognized that the symptoms you experience with your Crohn's disease – usually repeated bouts of diarrhoea containing blood and mucus – are very similar to those of infectious diseases of the bowel. Acute Crohn's disease can easily mimic cholera, and shigella can easily be mistaken for acute ulcerative colitis. The diseases are so similar in the way they affect people that past generations of doctors were convinced that both types of colitis were in fact infections from an as yet unknown germ, virus, bacterium or protozoon. Crohn's was even compared with tuberculosis of the bowel. Tuberculosis has thankfully become much rarer since all milk is pasteurized.

However, none of these searches for an infectious cause of Crohn's has ever been successful. That's a pity, because it would make treatment so much easier. It is curious, too, because the mucosal cells (see Chapter Three) in Crohn's disease often look just like the mucosa in a proven infection. What is certain is that the mucosa in Crohn's disease is the tissue that is affected, and that it is inflamed and damaged, even if not infected by any outside organism.

Perhaps this is the point at which we should consider the mucosa in a little more detail. In normal health, the cells in the mucosa of the small intestine, as mentioned in Chapter Three, must secrete mucus and be extremely active in pumping water and digested foodstuffs (the remnants of fats, proteins, sugars and starches, minerals and vitamins) across the barrier between the lumen and the body's internal circulation.

To do that, the cells are arranged in columns, several deep, and the mucosa itself is arranged in a myriad of folds and 'crypts' that are always moving and changing in shape. The constant movement and rippling ensures the maximum of contact between the contents the lumen and the surface of the mucosal cells. If anything happens to decrease that contact between contents and the healthy cells in the bowel surface, then water will remain inside the lumen and diarrhoea will surely follow.

The invention of the flexible fibre-optic endoscope lets us see exactly what is happening in all forms of bowel disease, and has been a huge boost to our knowledge of Crohn's and how it can be treated. Using endoscopy from above to look at the stomach and small bowel, and endoscopy from below to see the colon, specialist gastroenterologists and their surgical colleagues (they call themselves Digestive Endoscopists) are now able to see exactly what is happening in the chronically inflamed bowel.

They make their diagnoses in two ways. What they see in the bowel wall is often enough to help them make a provisional diagnosis, and the microscopic appearance of tiny pieces of tissue (biopsies) taken from the mucosa usually confirms their suspicions.

The normal bowel looks obviously healthy through the endoscope. What the endoscopist sees is the inner lining surface of the epithelium – the mucosal surface. It looks unbroken, glistening, smooth, with the odd blood vessel coursing along it. The folds, ridges and valleys are easily seen, and there is the occasional movement and ripple as the normal muscle movement in the wall carries on.

In Crohn's disease of the ileum there are patches of red, swollen mucosa, with obvious ulcers (breaks in the mucosal surface, much like large mouth ulcers) in the patches. Between the patches the rest of the bowel usually looks normal. The commonest area to be affected is the last few inches of the small bowel and the first part of the ascending colon, or the caecum. In some cases of Crohn's, the inflamed patches are also present in the rest of the colon, so that it is justifiable to call Crohn's disease a 'colitis' even though it largely affects the ileum, or small bowel.

Ulcerative colitis usually affects a different area of bowel from Crohn's. It does not spread into the small bowel, being confined to the colon. It tends first to affect the rectum and margin of the anus, where it is called proctitis, and then spreads upwards to the rest of the colon.

The two types of colitis differ in the extent to which they affect the bowel wall. While ulcerative colitis confines itself to attacking only the mucosa, leaving the outer layers of the bowel wall intact, Crohn's affects the whole thickness of the bowel wall. This can often lead to 'fissures' (cracks that extend through the wall of the bowel) and 'granulomas', which are masses of chronically inflamed tissue, much like internal boils. The experienced endoscopist can quickly tell the difference between the two through the endoscope, but will still need the pathologist's report of the extent and severity of the inflammation before making the final decision on diagnosis.

Common to both conditions under the microscope are masses of 'inflammatory' cells, identical to the white cells circulating in the blood. In normal tissues, they are few in number. In patches of Crohn's disease or in ulcerative colitis, they dominate the microscopic picture. The normal architecture of columns and ridges of healthy mucus-secreting cells has been replaced by a level surface in which the cells either appear flattened and empty, or are even absent altogether, being replaced by a mass of inflammation. In such areas where the mucosa has gone, there is no barrier between the contents of the lumen and the body's internal tissues and bloodstream. This is an obvious recipe for severe illness and toxicity.

Of course, not all that seems to be Crohn's or ulcerative colitis is necessarily one of them. Endoscopists have been caught by surprise, when what they thought before the examination would be a straightforward case has turned out to be much more complex. The biopsy may show an unexpected infection, or a rare type of bowel problem that mimics colitis. These will be covered later in the book. First, however, it is appropriate to devote a chapter each to Crohn's and to ulcerative colitis.

Chapter Five

Descriptions of Crohn's Disease

In May 1932, Dr Burrill Crohn of New York described what he believed was a new disease to his fellow physicians at a meeting in New Orleans. Patients with it, he said, had repeated attacks of diarrhoea, sometimes bloody, and he could feel a mass – a lump – in the lower right side of the abdomen. He had operated on 14 patients with this disease, and the mass turned out in each case to be a thickening and inflammation of the lower end of the small intestine, just before it became the colon. This was the 'terminal ileum' (the last part of the ileum) and he called the disease terminal ileitis.

He was careful to tell his colleagues that the mass was not a tumour – a cancer – nor was it a recognized infection. In particular, it was not tuberculosis of the bowel. Tuberculosis was, of course, much more common then than it is now.

Colleagues at the meeting respectfully suggested that he call it 'regional ileitis', as the word 'terminal' had overtones that might well be misunderstood by his patients! He agreed, not just because of the nuance of the meaning of 'terminal', but also because he had found in some patients patches of inflammation further up the ileum – so that it was truly regional, rather than just sited at the 'terminus' of the ileum. Others began to realize, as more cases were reported, that the disease could also spread into the colon, so that even the word 'ileitis' was not always accurate. Out of respect for Dr Crohn, the name 'Crohn's disease' started to be used, and it has stuck ever since.

However, that isn't the whole story. Professor Brooke, my old mentor, if he had his way, would have called it Dalziel's disease. Dr Kennedy Dalziel of Glasgow's Western Infirmary described it at a British Medical Association meeting in 1913, 19 years before Crohn's famous paper. He called it 'chronic interstitial enteritis' and described nine cases in his report. He pointed out that it affected other parts of the small intestine apart from the terminal ileum. Unfortunately his paper in the *British Medical Journal* of 1913 must have been missed by Professor Crohn and his colleagues. Perhaps the journal was not as prestigious in American eyes in the 1930s as it is now. Maybe it is just as well, as it is difficult to imagine doctors outside the UK pronouncing Dalziel's name correctly – for those not in the know, Dalziel is pronounced Dee-Yell.

Today we know Crohn's disease as primarily affecting young women, although it does occur in men, too. In Professor Crohn's time it was a rarity. For the last 30 years, all over the developed world, the numbers of cases have been climbing. Swedish doctors reported a rise from 2.5 to 10 cases per 100,000 people over the 19 years from 1955 to 1974.[1] In Scotland the figures for onset of Crohn's disease in people under 19 years old (about one-third of all cases start in childhood and teenage years) steadily increased from under 10 to 30 per million from 1968 to 1992.[2] The biggest increase was in the 12-16-year age group.

Whatever the exact numbers, it is clear that Crohn's disease is now widespread among our young people of both sexes. And it is a formidable enemy, producing not just bloody diarrhoea, but also many other symptoms.

It is not just confined to the gut. To begin at the 'top' of the digestive system, people with Crohn's (and, for that matter, those with ulcerative colitis) are more prone than others to repeated mouth ulcers, and microscopic examination of the surfaces inside the mouth reveals areas of inflammation that do not occur in people without Crohn's. Crohn's sufferers also show inflammation inside the stomach, in which there are often ulcers that look just like the mouth ulcers: there can be scarring and narrowing of parts of the stomach that resemble the picture seen in people with chronic bacterial infections of the stomach.

About 5 per cent of all people with Crohn's have a particularly severe infection, with patches of inflammation throughout the small bowel. This form of the disease is almost exclusive to teenagers; when the disease starts in the twenties and beyond, it is usually confined to the terminal ileum – the condition described by Professor Crohn in his original patients. In a minority of patients, Crohn's continues through the ileo-caecal valve into the colon, producing a true colitis, similar in its symptoms to ulcerative colitis. In a few cases only the anal region is involved.

Colonic Crohn's is more common in older men and women, particularly in those who have their symptoms for the first time after they are 60 years old. P J Fabricius and colleagues, following patients in Birmingham, found that around 8 per cent of their Crohn's patients were over 60 when first diagnosed (Fabricius, PJ et al. 'Crohn's disease in the elderly'. *Gut* 26(1985): 461-465). Half of them had the usual terminal ileum disease, some of which had extended into the right side of the colon, but in 40 per cent the disease was confined to the left side of the colon. These patches of inflammation may have been linked to diverticular disease, a very common problem for the elderly that is usually confined to the descending colon.

So far, what I have described is where the disease usually arises in various parts of the gut in people of different ages. To give an idea of the kinds of symptoms these different presentations of Crohn's produce, it is probably easiest to describe typical patients and what brings them to their doctors.

Emma was 12 when she was first taken to her doctor by her worried mother. She had had bouts of abdominal pain that her mother had thought were just stomach cramps, probably leading up to her first period. It was when the cramps were linked with repeated bouts of diarrhoea (at first attributed to 'nervousness'), coupled with the fact that she was becoming noticeably thinner, that her mother began to worry.

Her doctor noticed that she was quite small for her age, despite the fact that both parents were taller than average. And at 12 he would have expected the beginning of breast development: there was no sign of that. Her height turned out to be well below the fifth centile for her age (so that out of 100 girls of her age compared for height, she would be in the shortest five).

Feeling her abdomen, he felt a resistance to pressure in the area below and to the right of the navel. She complained that this area was tender to his touch, although she denied that she had any pain when she was sitting normally.

Putting the history together – the repeated diarrhoea, the failure to grow, the delayed puberty and the mass in the right lower quarter of the abdomen – her doctor suspected one of two diagnoses. The first was that she could have had a 'missed appendix' – an old appendicitis that had not been diagnosed in the past and had left her with a low-grade abscess. The second was Crohn's. Not really believing in a 'grumbling appendix' he opted for the second diagnosis, and asked for her to be seen by the local children's specialist gastroenterologist.

She arranged for Emma to have a small bowel barium enema, an X-ray in which barium is given to reach the ileo-caecal region. It showed the typical feature of Crohn's disease of that region – the 'string sign'. That area of gut looks just like a piece of string because it has been so narrowed by old scarring and current inflammation.

From then on the doctors knew what they were dealing with. Obviously the initial priority was to prevent her from having future bouts of pain and diarrhoea. But there was another priority: to improve her nutritional state and to help her make up for her lost growth and her delayed puberty. The most obvious way to do this was to give her first an 'elemental diet' to build up her lost proteins, fats and sugars, as well as vitamins and minerals, and then to remove the offending 'string' section of her ileum at operation. Surgery like this is only considered if the disease is confined to a single area, and there is good supporting evidence that it will lead to a dramatic improvement in a child's life. Emma had her operation and has not looked back since.

Professor M J G Farthing of St Barts' Hospital, London, wrote in 1992[3] that the most dramatic reversals of growth arrest have followed such surgery in children. He warned then against giving children like Emma prolonged steroid (cortisone-like) treatment, as this might curb growth even further.

Today we have steroid preparations that can be given with little risk of side effects to youngsters like Emma with Crohn's disease of the ileum and first part of the colon. The one that is licensed for this purpose in the United Kingdom is modified-release budesonide, given as a 3-milligram dose three times a day for eight weeks. The treatment stops after that time. The elemental diet is given in hospital, and can be carried on under the supervision of the family doctor's team at home. It isn't very pleasant to start with, but the fast improvement in the child's health makes it well worth persevering with until the bowel is no longer inflamed and can do the work of digestion itself. In the United Kingdom, the doctor can write the prescription for the diet – there are dozens of trade names for them – as long as the prescription is labelled ACBS and the reason for the diet (Crohn's disease) is kept in the records. ACBS stands for the Advisory Committee on Borderline Substances. These are medications that are not strictly drugs, but in this case foods, and that should be reserved for special cases like Crohn's and other digestive diseases.

Emma recovered well from her first episode of Crohn's, and has had no relapses since then. Her hospital doctors felt there was no need for long-term treatment to suppress future attacks, and so far they have been right. The long-term outlook for Emma today is very bright, with a good chance that the disease will die away and that she will grow up to a normal height and weight.

However, surgery for Crohn's disease is only for the few. If at all possible, gastroenterologists prefer to treat it medically. That's because the disease has the unfortunate tendency to return at the site of the old operation – in fact, at or just above the suture line where the two ends of the severed bowel have been joined. So when Andrew, aged 18, started to have severe bloody diarrhoea, surgery was not on the agenda.

Andrew was a student in his first year at university when the diarrhoea hit him for the first time. He had always been a 'faddy' eater, and at first he thought the diarrhoea had been a reaction to his poverty-stricken student's attempts at home cooking. However, the appearance of blood in the motions, and his realization that he was very much more ill than he would have expected from a normal stomach upset, made him call on the university doctor. She took no time at all in admitting him to hospital, as she immediately realized he was suffering from a severe bowel inflammation, probably peritonitis.

She had seen at once that he was ill. His eyes and cheeks were sunken, he was pale and clammy, and his abdomen was very tender to the touch – all over. When she pressed gently then released her hand, he had a short sharp spike of pain. He was very dry. When the doctor picked up a small fold of skin on the back of his hand, it did not immediately smooth back again to a level surface, but stayed there, in a ridge – a sign of considerable loss of body fluids.

Her only course was to send him to hospital, where the surgeons confirmed that he had 'acute diffuse small bowel Crohn's disease'. He was admitted to the emergency ward, where he was given intravenous fluids to replace the lost fluids and high doses of the cortisone-like steroid prednisolone, first by injection, then, as he improved, by mouth, to try to reduce the inflammation. He was also started on the antibacterial drug metronidazole, and samples of his stools were sent to the laboratory to identify any possible infection.

Over the next few days, Andrew gradually recovered. He was quickly rehydrated by the intravenous fluids, and started to feel better. His abdominal pain and diarrhoea subsided and he began to become mobile again. However, he was very weak for two or three weeks after this acute experience.

During this convalescent period, his university doctor and her hospital colleagues discussed his case. They were all concerned at his level of stress. He was struggling to feed himself on a wholly inadequate income, and was facing tough examinations. An intelligent and hardworking student, he was also very conscientious, and often studied alone late into the night. He was worried about his future, and his spell in hospital, he felt, was pushing him further back in his planned course of study. He was missing lectures, tutorials and practical sessions – and this was increasing his stress.

His doctors contacted his tutors, and it was agreed that he could take time out to recover his full health without prejudice to his eventual degree. This news was a big relief to him, and his physical improvement accelerated from then on. For his doctors, this relief from stress was just as important as the drugs and fluid replacement. It is difficult to study the effects of stress in humans with bowel disease, but there is very clear evidence in mice with a similar form of inflammatory bowel disease that stress brings on relapses in the condition.

There are good reasons for believing that the same happens in people. Psychological stress does directly affect mucosal cells, making them much more vulnerable to the passage of bacteria across their surfaces, from the lumen of the bowel to the tissues under the mucosa. There, they would meet up with the body's defensive system (about which more later) and trigger severe inflammatory reactions. Even if they do not cause bacterial peritonitis, these misplaced bacteria could easily cause an acute Crohn's episode in people who are susceptible to this type of reaction.

We are only now beginning to recognize that there are people like Emma and Andrew who are different, in that their defence systems can be stimulated into such reactions. More than that, the researchers are beginning to be able to identify them from genetic testing, and better still, they are beginning to produce drugs that will stop them happening. *Infliximab* is the first. *Thalidomide* – yes, the same drug that caused so much tragedy in the 1960s – is another. Many more will follow. How they work is explained in Chapter Six; how they can be used is shown in Anne's case below.

Anne was 19 when her diarrhoea started. She, like Andrew, fell ill quickly. She was hot and sweaty, with a lot of abdominal pain, and passed several bloody watery stools in a few hours. She felt sick all the time, and was unable to keep even a few sips of water down before retching and vomiting it back up. Her doctor admitted her to hospital as an emergency, and like Andrew she was given intravenous fluids, steroids and an antibiotic to try to return her to a normal, fully hydrated state.

In the beginning Anne responded reasonably well to this treatment. The good progress she made, however, came to a 'plateau'. After two weeks, although she felt better, she was still having troublesome and bloody diarrhoea. The antibiotic was stopped, and she was put on a 5-aminosalicylate, an anti-inflammatory drug that has been found useful in both ulcerative colitis and Crohn's.

Unfortunately, she did not respond to this treatment as completely as Andrew and Emma. Although she had improved from her acute, very ill state, she continued to have bloody diarrhoea, felt generally ill, and did not start to gain the expected weight. She became so weak and anaemic from the blood loss that she was given a blood transfusion, which produced an immediate improvement in her wellbeing, but still did not solve the problem of the continuing diarrhoea.

Worried that her recovery was too slow, Anne's specialist team decided to try an 'immune suppressant' drug. They considered a choice from three drugs: azathioprine, mercaptopurine and methotrexate. It wasn't an easy decision, because all three have been reported to help ease Crohn's disease that is unresponsive to steroids and fluid replacement. But they are not yet licensed for use in Crohn's, and all may produce serious side effects. They felt that probably the safest option was methotrexate, once weekly.

This produced a slight extra improvement, but even after another week she was still having bloody diarrhoea. This was when they decided to start infliximab.

Infliximab is a 'monoclonal antibody' that acts against a substance called tumour necrosis factor alpha, or TNF-α. What it is, and what it does, is described in more detail in Chapter Six, which explains the most modern thinking on the processes that produce Crohn's disease, and how these processes can be blocked so that they can be reversed to allow the bowel to recover. It is enough to state here that infliximab worked well. It was given by an intravenous infusion over two hours, and Anne began to feel better within a few days. She was given another infliximab infusion two weeks later, and then after a further four weeks. Over the next year she was given an infusion every eight weeks. Over that time, she had no further episodes of Crohn's, and has been keeping well.

Today, in the right hands – a clinic that specializes in helping people with the various forms of colitis – most young people with Crohn's do well. If they do not respond optimally to the first line of treatment, there are others that can be offered. The cases I have described are typical, so that if you have Crohn's you can be optimistic that your illness can be kept largely under control. And as you grow older, into your late twenties, you can be fairly confident that it will die away.

Why did you get it in the first place? That is more difficult to unravel – but I'll give it a shot in Chapter Six.

Chapter Six

Crohn's – Why and How

Crohn's disease is a disorder mediated by T lymphocytes which arises in genetically susceptible individuals as a result of a breakdown in the regulatory constraints on mucosal immune responses to enteric bacteria. (Professor Fergus Shanahan, University College, Cork, in the *Lancet*, 5 January 2002, p. 62)

Professor Shanahan's statement probably means little to you, but for doctors it explains a lot. So please don't let it put you off reading further. If you have Crohn's, this chapter explains why you have it and, better still, how this understanding will lead to research that will provide you with effective treatment. In this chapter I will try to put Professor Shanahan's views into plain English for the layman who is interested in colitis. It therefore has a reader's health warning. Much of what follows is complex, and if you have no scientific training you may find it hard going. So if you want to skip it for the time being and go on to the next chapter, which is more about perspectives on Crohn's disease and aspects of living that may provoke it, then do so. But take some time later to come back and read this chapter, as it gives you a scientific grounding on inflammatory bowel disease and why some people, but not others, develop it.

To begin at the beginning. We start off, at birth, with a small bowel in which there are no germs and that has had no food to bother it. After birth, the bowel first comes into contact with the proteins from the mother's milk – or if the mother has not breast fed, from the different proteins in various cow's milk preparations. At weaning, when solid foods are added, the bowel gets another shock, as these foods present the mucosal cells not only with a wide variety of digested food proteins, but also with a healthy dose of bacteria. These bacteria usually thrive only in the colon, but they can creep up into the last part of the ileum.

All these proteins are 'foreign' to the mucosal cells. In other words, they are not found normally within the human tissue. And when our tissues come into contact with foreign proteins, they often react with an 'inflammatory' response. Our breathing organs (our noses, throat and lungs) and our skin are very good at doing so. That's why we react so badly to dusts in the air or chemicals on our skin. The inflammatory response is a defence reaction mustered to destroy the foreign protein, and sometimes it can go overboard and cause allergies such as chronic rhinitis (a permanently irritated nose), asthma (wheeze) and eczema and dermatitis (rashes).

We can't afford to have this happen in our mucosa. We need to process the foreign proteins that we have swallowed without instigating the full inflammation response, because if we over-reacted to them we would not be able to digest them. Literally, we would starve. So the normal gut mucosal cells are extremely tolerant of foreign proteins.

Professor Shanahan puts his case beautifully. He writes: 'In healthy individuals, the intestinal mucosa is in a state of controlled physiological inflammation.' He looks upon the immune system in the gut wall as being on ready alert, sampling and interpreting the environment within the lumen. Its response to normal food proteins and to the normal, non-disease-producing bacteria is constrained, but it retains the ability to respond aggressively against potential disease-producing germs. In order for the mucosa to remain healthy, the cells must recognize and tolerate, without mounting destructive action against, proteins from digested food that must pass through them into the circulation. They must differentiate between the proteins from the 'normal' bacteria that live in our gut inoffensively and those that are from disease-producing organisms. The former are left to get on with life. Faced with the latter, the mucosal cells must be able to 'call up' the immune system to eliminate them. That means, in short, producing a defensive inflammatory reaction in the bowel wall.

Put simply, Crohn's disease happens when these protective systems fail. For Professor Shanahan, the crux of Crohn's is that the mucosal cells have lost their ability to tell the difference between the normal bacteria that inhabit our gut (and which protect against invading outsiders) and pathogens (germs that cause disease) like cholera, typhoid and salmonella. The result is that the bowel wall starts to produce an inflammatory reaction to the normal material within its lumen.

How does this happen? There is very strong evidence that Crohn's disease is inherited, and that the flaw stems from very specific genetic defects that cause the person to produce substances (they are called 'pro-inflammatory cytokines') that induce inflammation inappropriately.

We have known for a long time that there is an inherited element in Crohn's and in ulcerative colitis. Some ethnic groups, such as Ashkenazi Jews, have much higher rates of Crohn's than the rest of the populations in their countries, even when dietary differences are taken into consideration. Blood relatives are more likely than spouses of people with Crohn's to develop the disease. Nearly half of the identical twins of people with Crohn's, but only 4 per cent of non-identical twins, have it. Interestingly, relatives of people with Crohn's have an increased risk of both ulcerative colitis and Crohn's: yet it doesn't seem to work the other way. Relatives of people with ulcerative colitis have a higher risk of developing ulcerative colitis themselves, but not of developing Crohn's. The risk of developing any form of inflammatory bowel disease is higher for relatives of people with Crohn's than for relatives of people with ulcerative colitis, suggesting that the Crohn's inheritance link is more powerful.

Genetic screening has begun to provide the information we need on exactly how susceptibility to inflammatory bowel disease is passed on in our genes. We have 23 pairs of chromosomes on which there are thousands of genes that control our biochemistry, some of which control the way we mount an anti-inflammatory response to the challenge of germs and other foreign proteins. Thanks to our ever-advancing knowledge of how to identify abnormal genes, by 2002 gene abnormalities linked to cases of inflammatory bowel disease had been found in six different chromosomes – chromosomes 16, 12, 6, 14, 19 and 5, in order of their discovery. At or near all these sites were genes that control the production of 'cytokines', the substances that control our inflammatory response to bacteria.

This isn't the place to go into the biochemistry of such cytokines in detail, but one of them deserves a mention, if only to serve as an example. It was the first to be found, on chromosome 16.[1] It was a mutation in what is labelled the NOD2 gene (genes are usually labelled with three letters and a number). NOD2 proteins are found inside 'monocytes', which are defensive 'white' cells in the blood and in the tissue just under the mucosa. These proteins are the main detectors ('receptors') of signals from disease-producing bacteria. When the NOD2 within a cell 'senses' a bacterial product nearby, it activates the rest of the monocytes around it to rally against the bacteria and to produce 'nuclear factors' that start up the inflammatory response. Anything that goes wrong with the NOD2 gene will directly affect the body's response to foreign proteins inside the gut. Mutations that induce the cells to produce excessive nuclear factor in response to normal, non-'foreign' proteins have been found in 20 per cent of all cases of Crohn's. People with the usual, non-mutated form of NOD2 are much less likely to develop inflammatory bowel disease.

The other gene locations susceptible to a change that leads to Crohn's disease are all similarly close to, or identical with, sites that control the production of other aspects of the inflammatory process. Names to be bandied about are interleukins, interferon, major histocompatibility complexes (MHCs), T-cell receptors, thromboxane, intercellular adhesion molecules (ICAMs), colony stimulating factors (CSFs) and protein tyrosine kinases. There is no need to go into all these substances in detail, except to state that they are all produced by the body's immune system as essential elements in the normal functioning of the body's defences against bacterial infection. If any one of them malfunctions or is deficient, the natural tolerance of the gut towards food and normal bacterial proteins can be lost. It seems that in Crohn's disease one or more of these 'chemical defence agents' is either deficient or over-active.

This knowledge gives the researchers a chance to develop drugs that will correct the fault. The more we know about the faults that lead to the disease, the better chance we have of overcoming it.

Yet inheritance doesn't explain everything. If everything depended on inheritance, then every identical twin of a patient with Crohn's would have it, too. And if it were caused by a single gene problem, cases within families would be much easier to trace and to predict.

So what is the next piece in the puzzle? Not everyone with the genetic make-up that is commonest in Crohn's disease actually gets the disease. Something in their environment, possibly at a very early age, plays its part. Evidence for this comes from the steep increase, in the developed world, in numbers of people with Crohn's disease since the mid-twentieth century. And as developing countries have become more industrialized, they have followed suit. Why should this have happened?

Professor Shanahan explains it this way. In the past, when we were exposed to water supplies infested with worms and protozoa, we needed our mucosa to be very active against them. The genetic mutations that now give some people Crohn's disease were an advantage against these infections, in that they helped the mucosa to mount a very active attack upon them. This involves the mobilization from the bloodstream to the mucosa of T-cells, a type of white blood cell that targets and destroys foreign proteins and the organisms, whether they are worms or bacteria, that produce them.

There are two types of T-cell responses – they are called, unsurprisingly, T1 and T2. In most people, the T1 and T2 responses are finely balanced. In the person who develops Crohn's disease, the T1 response dominates. Normally when the T-cells have done their job and eradicated the foreign protein that they are programmed to attack, they then receive a signal (from those cytokines mentioned above) to commit suicide. This process is called by the scientists 'apoptosis'.

It's probably a good idea to look at apoptosis in a bit more depth here, before going on, because it is crucial to why some people go on to have chronic diarrhoeal disease, and most people don't. Apoptosis is a very important mechanism for all cells, from the moment of our conception to our deaths. In the womb, as we develop our human form from the single cell that we were at conception, we go through many stages. At one point we develop gills, just like fish. Being surplus to our future requirements, the cells that have formed the gills are instructed, via cytokines, to undergo apoptosis, and they die off. Their contents are then used by other cells that need to continue to grow. Our hands and feet start off webbed. The cells that form the webs also respond to the apoptosis message, so that our fingers and toes can operate independently.

Apoptosis is also vital to our fight against cancer. Whenever a cell undergoes a mutation so that it has the potential to become cancerous, it has an internal system that recognizes the change. This sets off the chemical instructions to become apoptotic, the cell dies off and the danger is allayed. Something similar happens to a T-cell that has been used to fight an infection. Once it has engulfed the invading organism and destroyed it, it too receives the instruction to undergo apoptosis. This is part of the normal T2 cell response. The aim of it, presumably, is to make sure that any foreign protein remaining inside the T-cell from bacteria or viruses is totally destroyed: apoptosis ensures that this happens.

So, in a normal response to infection, the T-cells are summoned to the infected area, battle against the 'invaders', destroy them, then, once the battle has ended, commit suicide. There are plenty of other T-cells ready to take their place. In the person at risk of Crohn's disease, however, the apoptosis message doesn't get through. By a cell mechanism too complex to describe here,[2] the T-cells that have been 'activated' against the bacterial invader just keep on destroying any proteins that are seen as foreign. As the mucosal cells are quietly getting on with their job of transporting food-derived proteins from lumen to the bloodstream, the activated T-cells see them, erroneously, as 'foreign' and therefore as their next target. That begins the mucosal destruction that ends in ulceration and the areas of Crohn's disease.

Does that mean that the first attack of Crohn's disease was initiated by an infection? It seems so. But it may have been so slight an infection that it produced no symptoms – just a microbiological 'blip'. It also explains why no infectious agent is found when people are admitted to hospital with an acute episode of Crohn's. By the time they are in hospital, any infection initiating the process that has led to the disease has been long gone. It arrived, initiated the activation of the T-cells, and was eradicated. The T-cells, however, stayed around to wreak their continuing destruction.

There is plenty of evidence that Crohn's is linked to an initial infection. It starts with studies of the bowel and the normal bacteria within it. There are colossal numbers of bacteria in the normal colon. It has been calculated that there are ten times as many bacteria in the colonic lumen as there are cells in the whole human body. As many as 400 different species of bacteria live within it, completely at home with us, their human hosts. They cause no symptoms, and may even be beneficial because they are formidable competitors to any newcomer that wants to come in and disturb things.

Some of these normal (commensal) bacteria may provoke a little inflammation in the mucosa even in healthy people: others, like the species lactobacillus and bifidobacterium, do not. They are exceptionally well tolerated, and even in Crohn's disease they do not stimulate the T-cell response. Lactobacilli and bifidobacteria are the germs that colonize the bowel first, with breast feeding. They are thought to be the main reason for the much lower rate of gastroenteritis in breast-fed than in bottle-fed babies.

The bowel's bacterial population is called the 'flora' by bacteriologists: this must be the most euphemistic title in science, considering the 'soil' in which the 'flowers' are growing. The flora changes after weaning, when E. coli usually becomes the dominant species. Some E. coli strains found in the gut of people with Crohn's have been shown to 'stick' to mucosal cells: such adherent qualities may well be linked with the activation of an immune response. Whether this is the initial infection that stimulates the process leading to Crohn's is still to be proven. What is true is that Crohn's doesn't start until after weaning. Whether it is the introduction of foreign food proteins or the change in the flora that starts off the process is still a matter of debate.

Quite a few recent findings link the flora to Crohn's. Studies in animals in which the flora can be manipulated from birth have shown that different flora (that is, flora in which the range of bacteria varies widely) change the way the mucosal cells develop and function. They may damage the integrity of the mucosal cells so that they are easily inflamed. In humans, the patches of Crohn's are mostly in regions of the small intestine, such as the terminal ileum, with the highest numbers of bacteria. During surgery the contents of the bowel are diverted away from the inflamed area in a 'by-pass' operation, so that the surface of the mucosa is no longer exposed to bacteria and the mucosa heals. The converse is also true. Areas of Crohn's inflammation tend to develop where there are areas of bowel through which the flow of contents is very slow (say, in loops or 'bulges' forming after previous surgery or alongside diverticuli in the colon). These are areas with very high bacterial counts.

Researchers have even induced areas of Crohn's in susceptible subjects by instilling bacterial material into previously non-inflamed loops of bowel. Needless to say, the people taking part in these experiments did so after the dangers were explained to them and gave their full consent. Interestingly, they also developed patches of Crohn's after food particles were placed in similar loops. Tests in people with Crohn's have shown that they put up a vigorous immune reaction, including T-cell activation and the production of a host of inflammation-producing cytokines, against many of the bacterial constituents of the normal bowel flora. People without Crohn's do not react against them.

The 'crunch' proof comes from animal experiments. There are laboratory animals with inflammatory bowel disease that is similar to Crohn's. Two groups of researchers, working independently, have shown that for them to develop the disease their bowel must first be colonized by the normal flora found in adult animals in their species. If their gut remains sterile (which is possible in laboratory conditions, in which all the food, the bedding and the whole environment is germ-free) they just do not get Crohn's.[3]

A third group indicated the mechanism at work. Dr Y Cong and colleagues took activated T-cells (that is, T-cells that have already been stimulated to produce inflammatory substances) from animals with active Crohn's disease and put them into animals that were not yet affected by it. They immediately developed the illness.

The T-cell experiment strongly supports Professor Stranahan's contention that not only is the cause of Crohn's to do with the bacteria in the gut, but the mechanism is closely linked to abnormal T-cells that are supposed to be the first line of defence against them.

If that is not enough evidence, there is a final clincher. When Crohn's disease is treated by changing the flora, so that the dominant bacterium is no longer an E. coli but a lactobacillus, the disease can heal, and as long as the new flora type is maintained it does not recur. This has been shown in humans, as well as in animals.[4]

So can all this new knowledge lead to better treatments for Crohn's disease? In one sense, it has already done so. Now that we know that the disease is almost certainly caused by an excessive inflammatory reaction to bacteria in the gut, we have plenty of targets at which to shoot. We have drugs in research that can individually block most of the chemical reactions in the body that lead up to the inflammatory activity – they are called the pro-inflammatory cascade. Early in this chapter I listed a series of 'cytokines' and other substances, such as interleukins, interferon, MHCs and CSFs, that are all involved in producing the Crohn's reaction. Once each of these was identified, scientists were able to devise molecules and then medicines involving these molecules that would oppose their actions.

The first of these to reach the prescription pad is infliximab. It targets the substance TNF-α mentioned earlier. TNF stands for 'tumour necrosis factor', and is one of the 'suicide-promoting' substances that helps to tell cancer cells to die. Exactly how infliximab works is not absolutely clear, but it does interfere with the pro-inflammatory cascade, thereby reducing the inflammation within the bowel wall. It also prevents white blood cells (mainly T-cells) from being attracted to the site of the inflammation, further reducing the inflammatory response, and particularly the T1 response mentioned above, in the tissues. It also seeks out mucosal cells already coated with TNF-a (and therefore abnormal) and promotes their apoptosis. It even stops the growth of new blood vessels into the inflamed tissue, further reducing the inflammation.

This combination of effects, all of which reduce inflammation in the gut, makes infliximab the first truly curative drug for Crohn's. The second is not far behind, and is a surprising one. It is thalidomide. Thalidomide was the medical horror story of the 1960s, when, given as a sleeping tablet to pregnant women, it damaged their babies. They were born with deformed and even absent limbs, and with internal organ problems. The drug was abandoned, and rightly so.

However, it came back into medical practice in the fight against leprosy, when it was found to be the only drug to help relieve and prevent the severe nerve damage sometimes caused by the drugs used to cure the disease. It was only recently found that thalidomide worked by blocking the action of TNF-α. It should work in just the same way as infliximab. Naturally, women taking thalidomide will be warned against becoming pregnant, and offered full contraceptive advice.

Infliximab, which targets TNF-α, is only the first aim for medicines to arrest and reverse Crohn's. A second that has already been reported in the medical journals is 'recombinant human granulocyte-macrophage colony-stimulating factor', or GM-CSF. Granulocytes and macrophages are types of white blood cells that are heavily involved in the normal immune system. GM-CSF stimulates their production. People with certain forms of human immune deficiency diseases, in which granulocytes and macrophages do not function normally, often develop an illness identical to Crohn's disease.

Noting this, American researchers B K Dieckgraefe and J R Korzenick used GM-CSF in 15 people with moderate to severe active Crohn's disease. They gave themselves daily injections, which they tolerated well, with only mild side effects, such as redness at the site of the injections. Within eight weeks, 12 of the 15 were very much better, and 8 were in complete remission. The quality of their lives vastly improved. Some needed repeat treatments 8 to 16 weeks after finishing the original course: they responded as well to the second treatment as to the first. The authors, writing in the Lancet of 9 November 2002,[5] admit that theirs was a small trial with no control group, but that their 80 per cent response was much greater than they would have expected. They asked for other teams to repeat their work in larger studies. We will have to wait for confirmation from them before being sure that this treatment works safely for most people, but the preliminary results give us very good grounds to hope that it will.

These new types of treatment are not the only way forward. Professor Shanahan sees a great future for what he calls 'manipulation of the intestinal flora'. It is based on the judgement, from very good evidence, that the inflammation of Crohn's is caused by contact with the normal flora, largely of E. coli strains. If that can be changed to a much less pro-inflammatory flora, in which bacteria like lactobacilli dominate, the disease should subside.

When this idea was first promoted, the best way to accomplish this was thought to be with antibiotics. Kill off the E. coli with a selective antibiotic, it was suggested, and the lactobacilli, which are not susceptible to it, will flourish. The antibacterial drug metronidazole, which does act against bacteria like E.coli, and not against lactobacilli, has therefore been used in this way.

However, this approach has its drawbacks. Bacteria can become resistant to antibacterial drugs, and that can lead to even worse infections in the long run and a relapse of the disease. In particular, some antibiotic treatments in inflammatory bowel disease have led to overgrowth with a particularly nasty germ called *Clostridium difficile* – the 'difficile' presumably meaning difficult to manage.

Professor Shanahan prefers a different approach. He favours 'seeding' the bowel with 'probiotics', rather than antibiotics. Probiotics are cultures of bacteria that do not induce the inflammatory response in the mucosa. So the lactobacilli and bifidobacteria mentioned above that colonize the guts of breast-fed babies are top candidates for this treatment. Interestingly, however, there are particular strains of E. coli that are also probiotic, and unlike their toxic cousins do not cause the mucosa to react to them. Other bacteria used in this way are enterococci. Cocci differ in shape from bacilli, being spherical rather than rods, but they are common enough inhabitants in everyone's gut.

Probiotics are given as food supplements on their own or with complex sugars called polysaccharides that provide their nutrient while they become established in the small intestine. They are certainly effective in ulcerative colitis (see Chapter Nine for more on ulcerative colitis): there is good hope that they will work in Crohn's as well, judging from results in animals with the disease.

A future use for probiotics will involve genetic engineering. Because of bad publicity in the press about mad scientists tampering with the stuff of life, people are naturally wary, and even suspicious, about the manipulation of genes in the laboratory. However, it is difficult to see a downside to this plan. In 2000, Dr L Steidler and colleagues 'engineered' a bacterium called *Lactococcus lactis* to produce a substance called IL-10, or interleukin-10. *Lactococcus lactis* is one of the 'safe' bacteria, like lactobacilli and bifidobacteria, that does not provoke an inflammatory reaction. IL-10, a cytokine found in mammals like ourselves, and not in bacteria, is a powerful blocker of the type of inflammation that occurs in Crohn's disease.

They then used the engineered lactococci as a probiotic, placing them in the stomach of mice with a bowel disease just like human Crohn's. The treatment worked: the mucosa became normal. The lactococci did not irritate or inflame the bowel, and they continued to produce IL-10, which 'cured' the inflammation that was already there.

Normally IL-10 has to be given by injection, and it has quite severe side effects (for example, it creates a flu-like illness). So it is not used in normal medical practice. By making a bacterium produce it in this way, it gets right to the site of the inflammation and injury, and should not enter the circulation in any sizeable quantity. That should avoid, or at the very least minimize, its side effects. As long as the bacteria survive in the gut, they will produce enough IL-10 to keep protecting it against episodes of Crohn's.

It is a brilliant idea, and I would bet on its being used widely by 2006. It will take until then to clear all the tests of safety and efficacy in humans.

Chapter Seven

Crohn's – Myths and Maybes

Now you are through Chapter Six, you can relax a little. This chapter is less technical, and you may feel it is more relevant to the way you live. It brings together many of the questions that people with Crohn's often ask, most of which revolve round whether something they have done has initiated their disease. Unfortunately we can't always give a straight answer. It isn't always possible to say that a particular aspect of your early life has definitely led to your Crohn's, but we can sometimes state that it has had a greater or lesser chance of doing so. Probably the best way to show this is to make this chapter a 'question and answer' session. So here goes.

Q   Did my early diet have something to do with my Crohn's? I wasn't breast fed and was weaned on to solids very early – around four months.

A   I can't count the number of studies that have tried to link early diet with later Crohn's. The first studies, in the 1960s, linked cow's milk with Crohn's, and by 1969 it was reported that when American troops with Crohn's were given combat rations containing no milk products, their illness dramatically improved.[1] Sadly these cases were just a series of uncontrolled case reports, and no one has been able to reproduce them in controlled trials since then. Other reports have implicated high intake of cornflakes in causing Crohn's, but these reports have been contradicted by others, and the cornflake story is no longer believed.

However, the cornflake story may have been truer than we think. Several German studies in the 1970s, followed up in the 1980s in the United Kingdom, Israel and Sweden, have repeatedly implicated refined sugar. The more sugar you eat in childhood, the greater your chance of developing Crohn's in your teens and twenties. Of course, cornflakes contain a lot of sugar, and many people add more sugar to them, so that the cornflake link may have been a mistake. The real culprit in these trials may have been the sugar eaten along with them.

Why should sugar be a problem? There are two explanations: the sugar may have encouraged the more aggressive and pro-inflammatory bacteria to thrive (see Chapter Six). Or the high levels of sugars in the gut may have directly affected the mucosal cells' ability to cope with bacterial or food proteins. Either way it seems sensible for anyone with Crohn's to curb their refined sugar intake, and to do the same for children in the family. Remember that Crohn's disease is up to 30 times more common in first-degree relatives (sons, daughters, brothers, sisters) of people with the disease.

As for weaning too early or too late, the jury is out on that one. There are conflicting stories, mostly anecdotal, but no statistically confirmed proof that either early weaning or later weaning has any influence on later Crohn's disease. We do know, however, that Crohn's only develops after weaning, at whatever age.

Q   My daughter was always difficult to feed. She was very faddy as a toddler, and virtually lived on beans and chips until she was a teenager. She would always refuse other foods, like fruit and green vegetables. Is this faddiness part of the reason she developed Crohn's, and could she have avoided it if I had insisted earlier on a wider variety of foods in her diet?

A   This is a really difficult one to answer. One theory is that after weaning children should be given as wide a variety of foods as possible well before the age of two. This gives the mucosa plenty of time to become accustomed to, and tolerate, the different foreign proteins being presented to it before the immune system is fully established. Foods experienced before the second birthday should then not cause an inflammatory reaction after that age. However, if the child's gut is exposed to a very restricted diet before two, then any new food eaten for the first time after that age could provoke inflammation in susceptible people. However, this is theory, and remains a theory until someone can prove it. That will be difficult.

Another explanation for her faddiness may be that she sticks to foods that don't give her stomach pains: in other words, even at a very early age, normal foods may start to upset the mucosa. In that case, she will develop Crohn's in the long run, regardless of the food she ate as a toddler. My own gut feeling (no pun intended) is that children should be exposed to as wide a variety of foods as possible as soon as they are fully weaned from the breast. And for prevention of Crohn's breast does seem to be best.

As for her eating only beans and chips, the lack of fresh fruit and vegetables may have had a bearing on her illness. As long ago as 1987 an international study showed that people with Crohn's or ulcerative colitis had eaten, as children, substantially less fruit and vegetables than people of the same age and in the same environment with no inflammatory bowel disease.[2] Don't feel guilty about it: faddy eaters often put great pressure on their parents, who have a really tough time with them. But warn your daughter that when she has children she should ensure that her children eat well. Firmness is the name of the game.

Q   My daughter started smoking at 14. She had her first bout of Crohn's a few months later, just after her 15th birthday. Are the two connected?

A   Quite probably. Many studies in the 1980s showed conclusively that Crohn's is about four times more common in smokers than non-smokers. Probably the most relevant for the United Kingdom were those of the Royal College of General Practitioners Oral Contraceptive Study (RCGPOCS) and the Oxford Family Planning Study, two very large studies that showed that, in women, smoking was closely linked to the onset of Crohn's.[3] If your daughter wants to reduce the chances of future attacks she must stop smoking. The risk falls in ex-smokers.

Strangely, smoking is one habit that differentiates people with Crohn's from those with ulcerative colitis. People with ulcerative colitis tend to be non-smokers or ex-smokers. This was an astonishing finding of a huge study of 304,000 people in Washington State, USA, in which smokers had around 60 per cent of the risk of non-smokers (i.e. people who had never smoked) of developing ulcerative colitis.[4] More amazingly, smokers who had stopped had twice the risk of non-smokers of having ulcerative colitis. It seems that if you stop smoking, some change in your large bowel can precipitate ulcerative colitis. This is backed by the fact that the rate of ulcerative colitis in British and Irish Mormons, who don't smoke, is three times that of the overall population in their countries.[5]

I must say these figures are disquieting. I don't know of any other disease in which smoking offers clear benefits, and I would not advise anyone to start smoking to settle his or her ulcerative colitis, because smoking has so many other life-threatening consequences. But the fact that something in tobacco smoke may protect against ulcerative colitis may lead to new treatments for it.

However, this is certainly not the case for people with Crohn's. They should not smoke. For them stopping smoking could well reverse an acute attack and improve their health if their disease is 'grumbling on'. If you are a smoker and find it difficult to stop, then read the appendix on stopping smoking, the purpose of which is to provide you with the incentive to give up for good.

Q   My daughter has chronic Crohn's disease and is in a steady relationship. She feels that her general health is too poor for her to become pregnant or to look after a baby, and would like to use the contraceptive pill. She has heard, however, that the pill may make her worse. Is that correct? At the moment her partner is using condoms, which is unsatisfactory. She would like to start a family in the future, when she hopes to be much better physically than she is now. What should she do?

A   Here, too, there is no straightforward answer. Several early studies suggested that women using the contraceptive pill were twice as likely to develop Crohn's than non-users. However, the RCGPOCS study mentioned above cast doubt on this: it failed to show a significant difference. The original trials had looked at the use of the older pill types, and the risk rose the longer the women had taken the pill. It was not an immediate reaction. My own feeling is that she could try taking the pill under the supervision of her GP and consultant, and stop it if she feels she is getting worse. I am sure she is right to postpone pregnancy until she is physically fit and is in a complete remission (without any symptoms) from her disease. She can be encouraged that with modern treatment she has a very good chance of achieving such a state.

Q   I have Crohn's disease, and have a small hole in the right side of my abdomen that sometimes oozes fluids that make my skin raw and sore. I'm told that it is a fistula. What is this? Why can't the surgeons operate on it to close it? I'm told I'm to go on infliximab for it. Will that help?

A   Fistulas appear in around one-third of people with long-term Crohn's disease. They are the result of erosion of an inflammatory ulcer through the bowel wall, and then through your abdominal wall to the skin. It is in effect a tube carrying the fluid from your bowel to the outside. The skin soreness is because the fluid contains digestive juices. Fistulas can form between one part of the bowel and another, or to the skin, as in your case, or even from the bowel to the bladder. Surgery doesn't help because a new fistula often arises along the track of the operation.

  Happily, there is very good evidence that infliximab will help the fistula to heal. In an American study of 94 adults with several fistulas that had been present for at least three months, infliximab closed all the fistulas in more than half the patients, and closed more than half of the fistulas in more than two-thirds of the patients.[6] The benefit of the treatment was obvious within two weeks, and the fistulas remained healed for the following three months. So you have a good chance of doing well. And if the fistula persists, there should soon be even newer treatments for you, like the GM-CSF treatment mentioned in the previous chapter.

Q I have arthritis and eye inflammation as well as Crohn's. Are they all connected, or have I just had very bad luck in having three separate diseases?

A They are probably connected, and linked with an inherited problem that has given you difficulties in controlling inflammation. This means that much of the tissue in direct contact with the outside world, such as your skin, the surface of your eyes and the mouth and throat, tends to over-react. This leads to a chronic inflammation in the tissue, just as it does in your small intestine. So a small proportion of people with Crohn's also have inflamed eyes. When the whites of the eyes are involved it is called episcleritis, and when the iris is inflamed it is iridocyclitis. Many people with Crohn's have mouth ulcers, and some develop skin rashes in the form of raised red lumps on the lower legs, called erythema nodosum. Pyoderma gangrenosum is another, thankfully rare, skin condition that can complicate Crohn's. Although this sounds awful, it usually responds well to high doses of steroids.

Arthritis is also more common than usual in people with Crohn's. One particular form of it, ankylosing spondylitis, affects one in 100 people with either ulcerative colitis or Crohn's, in comparison with one in 10,000 people with no bowel disorder. Why the two should be connected is not known.

So you have been unlucky. But you can be reassured that much research is continuing into all these conditions and why they co-exist in some people. And that should lead to better treatments in the near future.

Q I am worried I will develop cancer. I have Crohn's, and a nursing friend tells me that people with Crohn's or ulcerative colitis have a higher chance than most of developing cancer. Is this true?

A Some friend, to make you worry in this way! Studies in the 1970s did show that people with Crohn's had a higher than normal risk of developing cancer. The cancers arose near the sites of inflammation in the gut and in organs distant from the gut. At that time it was estimated that 2.8 per cent of people with Crohn's might develop cancer over a period of 20 years.[7] Although this doesn't sound many, it is a rate 20 times that of the rest of the population. However, by 1981 a report from Birmingham brought this down to twice the normal rate.[8]

In the latest report to date (in 2002), 573 people with severe Crohn's that had not responded to the usual treatments were given infliximab.[9] Because they were being given a new drug, they were followed very carefully for possible side effects, which of course might include cancer. Six patients developed cancer during the follow-up. The cancer were all in different sites. Two patients developed different types of skin cancer, there was one kidney cancer, one bladder cancer, one breast cancer and one lymphoma. There were no bowel cancers, and no cancers at any site of Crohn's inflammation. This is a 1 per cent cancer rate in a group of chronically ill people: it is fairly similar to the rate that would be found in the general population. It would be difficult to prove that any of these cancers, except perhaps for the lymphoma, was caused by having Crohn's disease or the treatment for it.

At the very worst, the figures suggest that, if there is a higher risk of cancer in people with Crohn's, it only affects a very small minority of them. I'd make two further points. The first is that since treatments became more effective, people with Crohn's have had very much less time with active disease. As any cancer would be related to the severity and duration of the disease, the cancer risks reported in the 1970s should be much lower now. The second is that as people with Crohn's are in long-term follow-up from their doctors and their specialist clinics, any early sign of cancer should be picked up early enough for there to be a good chance of cure. So don't worry about something that may never happen, and get on with enjoying your life.

Q   Can a food allergy cause Crohn's? Whenever I have eaten bread I start to have stomach pains and pass blood in my motions. Should I have allergy tests?

A   A few people with Crohn's do seem to react badly to particular items in their diet. Wheat flour is the commonest culprit, followed by dairy products, green vegetables, maize and tomatoes. Lower down the list come citrus fruits, eggs, coffee, banana, meats, potatoes, rice, tea, fish, shellfish, chicken and chocolate. In fact, you name the food and someone with Crohn's has complained about it. However, people with Crohn's do not show the allergic response in tests. Technically, this means that they do not have the classical 'IgE' reaction (that, say, people with asthma and eczema have) which proves that they are allergic to the foodstuffs about which they complain.

So it is almost certain that you do not have a food allergy. However, if you do react badly to bread, then avoid it. You might like to try breads and biscuits that do not contain wheat instead. You may be reacting to the wheat flour, and be able to eat oats, maize, rye, chickpea or soya flour with no trouble.

Because what you can and can't eat is so important in any form of colitis, the next chapter is devoted to it.

Chapter Eight

Eating with Inflammatory Bowel Disease – Tackling Food Intolerance

I explained at the end of Chapter Seven that Crohn's is not an allergy in the true sense of the word. But that doesn't rule out the possibility that you may be intolerant of certain foods – that your mucosa reacts badly to them, without being involved in a full allergic reaction. The difficulty lies in proving that it does.

To prove that a particular food stimulates your Crohn's into activity, the most appropriate test is to wait until you have no symptoms and are in a remission, then give the food, and wait. Not surprisingly, not many people are willing to do that.

The brave Crohn's sufferers who do volunteer for studies into food-induced relapses have helped to clarify things a lot. To start with, some tend to react dramatically and immediately to a single 'challenge' with a small amount of a particular food protein. Others need to have several 'challenges' over a week before they begin to react against it with pain and diarrhoea.

The main difficulty has been in disguising the food under study. For a proper scientific study, the patient must not know what food he is being given, or whether in fact he is being given placebo instead of the food. The doctors giving the food mustn't know, either, so that the samples must be encoded and the key to the code (which states whether the sample is the food or a placebo) must be kept by someone not directly involved with the patient. Obviously the subject must not be able to taste the food either, as then the secret would be out. For a trial to be completely without bias, any psychological reaction to the taste must be ruled out.

Early trials used lentil soup as a disguise – it was assumed that the taste of anything added to it would be drowned by the strong lentil flavour. They had inconsistent results, largely because the soup tasted disgusting and the patients couldn't tolerate it for more than a day or two! The researchers then put the study foods into blackcurrant drinks that could be tolerated for seven days, and were still strong enough to disguise other tastes. In other, much less comfortable, trials subjects were asked to receive their test foods through a tube passed through their noses into their stomachs – 'nasogastric' tubes – thereby avoiding the taste problem.

The results of all these tests? There was no evidence of any allergy to food in people with Crohn's. Their disease did not re-activate on presenting any foods to their stomachs, in any of these trial systems. Interestingly, the same systems did find a lot of intolerance to various foods in people with irritable bowel. That's another story, to be explained in a following chapter.

So why is it that people with Crohn's so often complain that a particular food produces symptoms? One theory is that it provides nutrient for bacteria in the gut, which then can multiply and produce the pro-inflammatory reaction described in the previous chapter. It is your particular flora, almost unique to you, that holds the key to whether you are healthy or in relapse. The integrity of your mucosa may depend on your not cultivating a particular strain of bacterium in the lumen – and that may depend on whether or not it has a particular food protein on which to dine.

The proof of this has come from studies of the use of elemental diets to treat acute Crohn's disease. I touched on them before, in Chapter Five. Now is the time to go into them in detail.

Elemental diets are manufactured products, to be taken by mouth, that contain all the nutrients you need in their most basic forms. The food that we normally eat consists of fats, proteins, starches and sugars. In order to be able to use these substances ourselves, the gut has first to digest them – to break them down into their basic 'building blocks' – before we can then build them up again (mainly in the liver) into the fats, proteins and glucose that we need. Our mucosal cells have to work to make digestion happen. In Crohn's disease, many of them have already been destroyed in the inflammatory process, and many others are struggling to function. So if we take the strain off the mucosa by providing 'already digested' food materials, in theory they should be helped to recover.

So elemental diets contain the building blocks. Instead of fats, they contain fatty acids. Instead of proteins, they contain amino-acids and peptides. Instead of starches and sugars, they contain glucose. They also contain the correct proportions of the right minerals and vitamins. Probably the main ingredients in such elemental diets are the amino-acids. They are the substitute for proteins. Having read this far, you will know that it is proteins (whether from bacteria or from foods) that are responsible for the inflammatory reaction in the mucosa that leads to bouts of Crohn's.

The theory seems unarguable, but what happens in practice? The facts are unassailable. After two to four weeks of treating with elemental diets, 90 per cent of all patients with acute Crohn's get better. In medical terms they go into remission. They lose their abdominal pain and diarrhoea, they put on weight and they feel much better. Not only that, but the blood tests that showed they were in the grip of severe inflammation (they are called the ESR and C-reactive protein) also improve substantially.

The improvement people feel when they are on the elemental diet is not just because their nutritional state is better. Their mucosal cells also start to work normally again, so that they are no longer leaking fluid and white cells into the lumen. There is good evidence that on the diet the mucosa as a whole recovers and the ulcers and abscesses heal.

So far, so good. But there is a considerable downside to elemental diets. They taste terrible, so that people taking them need a lot of encouragement to keep on with them. For some people the only way to take them is by the nasogastric tube mentioned above. So they are not a permanent answer. Sadly, once people stop their elemental diet and return to normal eating, the disease recurs – in medical terms, they relapse.

If this is your problem, is there a way to eat normally again? Yes, but it is difficult to manage, and you need a lot of patience. The groundwork on how to do this was laid down as long ago as 1984, by Dr E Workman and colleagues.[2] They showed that people who have become normal, without symptoms, on an elemental diet can start slowly to return to a normal diet, adding new foods one by one over many weeks. If, after a new food is introduced the pain, and diarrhoea return, that food is permanently avoided. Doing this, seven out of every ten people whose Crohn's had been put into remission by elemental diet kept completely free of relapses, simply by avoiding foods that upset them. They didn't find it to difficult to keep up. This was a considerable contrast to the 'control' group of patients, who had also become symptom-free on the same elemental diet. They were put on a normal diet: eight out of ten had relapsed inside two months, and all had active Crohn's within six months.

It isn't easy to find the self-discipline to organize your diet in this way, but once you have recognized the big difference it can make to your life, you should be able to do it. In Dr Workman's study, there was no one food to be avoided. Different people found different foods upset them. The commonest were cereals and dairy products, but some people reacted to rice, barley or rye, or even to beef, turkey, turnips or onions. This differentiates Crohn's from coeliac disease, which is caused by intolerance to gluten (found in wheat flour,) and for which the universal cure in every patient is the complete avoidance of even the most minute quantities of gluten.

The good news is that it was rare for people with Crohn's to find that they were sensitive to a host of foods. Most reacted badly to only one or two foods, so that the exclusions were few and they could still enjoy a wide range of tasty and satisfying meals. Also unlike coeliac disease, if the person with Crohn's ate a small portion of their particular offending food by mistake, it did not cause them trouble. It needed a substantial helping to initiate symptoms. So the odd error did not lead to catastrophe.

If you succeed in finding the foods that upset you, and stick strictly to avoiding them, it is odds on that you will do well. Writing in 1991, seven years after first publishing their work on exclusion diets, members of the team reported that the improvement in the health of the patients who stuck to their diets was maintained. Two years later, two-thirds of them had had no recurrences, and around half continued to remain well on the diet alone four years later. Several more were doing well on the exclusion diet plus a small regular dose of steroids.

Those who can't stick to the exclusion diet, or who find that they must exclude too many items of food to make it practical, need extra help. This may be available to them in the drug treatments mentioned in Chapter Five. They also may have the choice of a 'formula' diet, which is somewhere between an elemental diet and normal food.

Elemental diets were described earlier in this chapter as the building blocks of our food. Formula diets are a little more complex. Instead of fatty acids and amino-acids, they contain more complex fats (triglycerides), fibre and peptides. In theory, even though they are more complex molecules, they should be less likely to stir up an inflammatory response in the mucosa than the normal proteins and fats in food. The fact that they are more complex than elemental diets makes them more palatable, so that they can be swallowed rather than delivered by tube. They also cost much less, which is important when they have to be used long term.

Formula diets may be offered to any Crohn's patient who needs them, particularly if the symptoms are continuing despite the standard treatment, and an exclusion diet hasn't worked or has been impossible. They are particularly useful in building up strength in people who have been weakened by their constant diarrhoea and pain, and who find that normal food is not helping them. Underweight and under-height children are good candidates for formula diets, and so are pregnant women with active Crohn's. Newborn babies of mothers with active Crohn's treated with formula diets have been reported to be of normal weight and healthy.

Formula diets are usually started in hospital, to give the patient time to get used to them. It isn't just a matter of giving you the packages and telling you to 'get on with it'. You need training in the management of home nutrition, and it can take several days to organize it and to feel comfortable with it. People with Crohn's, however, seem to be more motivated than most to accept awkward treatments. I don't find this a surprise. They will put up with a lot to end the cycle of constant stomach discomfort and diarrhoea, with the inevitable weakness and tiredness they bring.

Much the same applies to people with ulcerative colitis, which although it causes similar symptoms is a very different disease, with different treatments and complications. It is the subject of the next four chapters.

Chapter Nine

Ulcerative Colitis – A Background

Unlike Crohn's, which mainly affects the small intestine, ulcerative colitis limits itself to the colon, the large intestine. Medical students are taught that it takes three forms: mucous colitis, relapsing colitis and fulminant colitis. The first is the least worrying in the short term. It is less severe than the other forms, and the patient has repeated attacks of diarrhoea in which there is an abundance of mucus and some blood.

In relapsing colitis the disease is more 'aggressive'. There is a chronic active state of bloody diarrhoea, in which the colon becomes progressively more ulcerated. The colonic mucosa reacts by thickening and growing fleshy lumps, called pseudopolyps, that grow into the lumen. In its final stages, the colon wall becomes thinner and smoother – in medical parlance 'atrophied'. This atrophic colonic lining is very susceptible to becoming cancerous.

Fulminant colitis is life-threatening. The colon swells, balloon-like, and stops working. The patient becomes very toxic, with a fast heartbeat, fever and a swollen and very tender abdomen. The diarrhoea that the patient has had in the days beforehand stops as the bowel becomes paralysed. If it is not treated urgently, the bowel wall disintegrates and the patient dies from peritonitis and septicaemia. The usual treatment is an emergency removal of the whole colon – a colectomy.

The aim of management of ulcerative colitis is to prevent mucous colitis and relapsing colitis from becoming fulminant. If that can't be prevented, then surgery is inevitable. Today, after such surgery, most people with ulcerative colitis recover quickly and enjoy a normal life. How doctors and patients with ulcerative colitis can work together to achieve this is the subject of the next four chapters.

First, a bit of history. I was impressed to find, on doing my research for this book, that Bonnie Prince Charlie had a role to play in the treatment of ulcerative colitis. He cured himself of what he called a 'bloody flux' by excluding all milk from his diet. Being a patriotic Scot myself, I wasn't too sure what to make of this information. He's not my favourite man. In fact, if my ancestors were at Culloden they were probably fighting against him. So, if he was responsible for one of the ways to treat ulcerative colitis, this was his only redeeming feature in my eyes.

Charlie's bloody flux was almost certainly an attack of ulcerative colitis. It is not a new disease. And it is widespread. It affects people all over the world, and so has attracted the attention of medical number-gatherers from almost every country. That is how we know that it affects around 10 per 100,000 people per year in most countries. It is less common in eastern and southern than in northern and western Europe. In the United States it was reported to affect farmers much less often than townspeople, a finding since repeated in Germany, Italy, Scotland and Finland, but not, apparently, in Oxford. Perhaps Oxfordshire farmers are more urban, or perhaps more genteel, than they care to think.

It does run in families, but it appears that inheritance in ulcerative colitis is not as important as it is in Crohn's. The incidence of identical twins who both have ulcerative colitis is much lower than that in Crohn's. When 152 patients with ulcerative colitis were compared with the same number of people without it from the same social class, eight relatives of the cases, but only one relative of the controls, also had the disease. If the same had been done for Crohn's, the expected figure for the relatives of the cases would have been around 30.

So it seems that the environment is more important than genetics in initiating ulcerative colitis. Here comes Charles Edward Stuart again. The milk story was spot on. Milk-free diets have been promoted for patients with ulcerative colitis since the early years of the twentieth century.[1] In 1961, S C Truelove was writing in the *British Medical Journal* about 'Ulcerative colitis provoked by milk'.[2] Several reports link later ulcerative colitis to lack of breast feeding in the newborn and the early substitution of cow's milk. J F Mayberry, writing in 1991, stresses that 'a period of breast feeding as short as two weeks may reduce the risk of ulcerative colitis in later life.[3]

The real puzzle about ulcerative colitis, however, is its relationship with smoking. It was mentioned in Chapter Eight, in relationship to Crohn's, but it is worth repeating again here. In probably the most extensive study of the lifestyles of people with inflammatory bowel disease, the relative risk of developing ulcerative colitis in ex-smokers who had previously smoked heavily was four.[4] This means that, proportionately, 4.4 times as many people in this group had ulcerative colitis than the average of the whole population studied. The corresponding figures for all ex-smokers was 2.5, for non-smokers 1.0 and for current smokers 0.6. These astonishing figures suggest that by smoking people cut their chances of developing ulcerative colitis by 40 per cent.

Why this should be could be a major pointer to the causes of ulcerative colitis. Smoking is known to increase the mucus production in the colon, just as it does in the lung. It is known to alter immune reactions. And it slows down the muscular activity in the colon wall. It also reduces the production of two inflammatory cytokines – they are called interleukin-1ß and interleukin-8. And it tends to block the action of T2, but not T1 cells. All these are processes that are important in initiating and maintaining inflammation in the colon mucosa.

So the colon seems to be topsy-turvy. Smoking normally irritates organs and causes inflammation. In the colon it seems to prevent it. The same goes for 'non-steroidal anti-inflammatory drugs' or NSAIDs. These are the anti-arthritic and pain-killing drugs everyone takes nowadays for colds and aches and pains. Examples are ibuprofen, indomethacin, naproxen and aspirin. Not only do they not soothe an ulcerated colon, they can make it worse. There have even been reports that they can initiate the disease.[5]

After doubts had been cast on the role of the oral contraceptive pill in causing ulcerative colitis, it has been exonerated by a large Italian trial which showed that it was not linked with any significant risk.

Forty per cent of people with repeated attacks of ulcerative colitis say that psychological stress can cause them. Longer-term stress, such as worries about work or studies, or marital or money worries, are more likely to cause the illness than shorter-term anxiety, as with a row. This is backed up by animal studies in which long-term stress causes the colon to produce less mucus and causes the colonic mucosa to become more permeable to bacterial proteins.

The bacterial story may be quite important. The strongest protection of all against developing ulcerative colitis is to have your appendix out early in childhood, and certainly before you are 20 years old.[6] It seems that some infectious agent not yet identified, or some bacterial antigen (an antigen is an inflammation-promoting protein on the surface of a bacterium or virus), lurks in the appendix perhaps long after the germ has gone. There is one caveat to the appendix story: the operation has to have been for confirmed appendicitis or for a related infection, mesenteric adenitis, if its removal is to protect the patient. If your appendix is removed incidentally while you are having an operation for another problem, such as a hernia, then you will not be protected – you have the same risk as someone who still has his or her appendix.

This has two possible explanations. Having an inflamed appendix, or inflammation of the lymph glands beside the appendix, may protect against later ulcerative colitis. So it may not be the removal of the appendix itself that helps, but the inflammation that provoked the appendicitis in the first place. The other explanation is that a genetic tendency towards having ulcerative colitis may protect you against developing appendicitis. Interpreting medical facts isn't always straightforward!

Which leads us to the role of bacteria in the gut as causes of ulcerative colitis. If you have read the chapter on Crohn's you will realize by now how complex that can be. The first piece of evidence that bacteria play their part in causing ulcerative colitis comes from laboratory animals. There are strains of animals that are prone to ulcerative colitis, with the same pattern of disease as humans. They do not develop it if they are kept in a germ-free environment and their food is always sterile. As soon as they are exposed to the normal flora that inhabit the gut in animals of the same species, they develop ulcerative colitis. If at the same time they are given antibiotics to suppress the bacteria, their ulcerative colitis is not nearly so severe as it is without the antibiotics.

The second main piece of evidence is that ulcerative colitis starts in the sigmoid colon and rectum – near the end of the colon, where there are the most bacteria. With time, it spreads upwards into the ascending colon: the extent and severity of the disease mirrors the gradient of the numbers of bacteria in that part of the colon. The more the bacteria, the more severe is the disease.

The third piece of evidence comes from the colonic mucosa. Analysis of colonic mucosal cells and their reactions to bacteria shows that they are unable to distinguish between the antigens on the surface of 'normal' commensal bacteria and those on the surface of disease-producing bacteria. They react with an inflammatory reaction to both equally. This is quite different from the reactions of mucosal cells from people without ulcerative colitis. In other words, they are no longer tolerant of harmless colonic flora. They see harmless bacteroides bacteria, which inhabit the lower colon of all of us, as potentially dangerous 'pathogens' (bacteria that cause disease). And they react accordingly by mounting an inflammatory 'challenge' to them that leads to ulceration.

Why should the colonic mucosa act in this way? As with Crohn's disease, the researchers have identified faulty genes in people that are strongly linked with ulcerative colitis. However, they are on different chromosomes (3, 7 and 12) from those linked to Crohn's.

The cytokine story explained in the section on Crohn's also applies to ulcerative colitis – but again, the details differ. In ulcerative colitis there are changes in different interleukins and in different T-cells, so that treatments for it to be developed on the basis of blocking cytokines may need to be different from those for Crohn's. In the meantime, we have to make do with the current treatments, improvements in which, over the years, have been gradual but relatively successful.

Chapter Ten

Current and Future Treatments for Ulcerative Colitis

Treatment for ulcerative colitis is divided into induction therapy for bringing about remission of the acute disease and then maintenance therapy to keep it from recurring. They need quite different approaches.

The first priority for anyone with an acute attack of ulcerative colitis is to be admitted to hospital and to be given enough of the right sort of drug in the right way to be sure that the acute inflammation is reversed as soon as possible. In the meantime, fluids must be given to counter dehydration. Often they must be given intravenously.

The drug of first choice for mild to moderate active ulcerative colitis is an aminosalicylate, mesalazine. It is given by mouth or as an enema, particularly when the site of the ulceration is in the lower colon and rectum. Often it is given by both routes. This initial period of high-dose mesalazine lasts for four to six weeks before the next phase, steroid treatment, is considered.

Until recently the choice steroid was prednisolone. It has been replaced by budesonide, which has the advantage of being highly active on the mucosa in the colon, but being broken down as it passes through the liver, so that it does not reach the general circulation in a significant amount. This means that it gives far fewer and much less serious side effects than other steroids, while doing its job at the site of the inflammation. Budesonide, prednisolone and mesalazine can all be given by enema, so that the consultant in charge has a choice of treatments to offer.

Unfortunately, some people with acute ulcerative colitis do not respond completely to the first-line treatments. If the bleeding and diarrhoea continue to cause poor health, the physician's next drug of choice may be ciclosporin, given by intravenous drip. Three trials have shown that it induces remission in between 60 and 80 per cent of people with severe acute ulcerative colitis.[1]

However, ciclosporin must be given with great care, as it can occasionally reduce the activity of the immune system to such an extent that the patient can be overwhelmed by what would otherwise be a mild infection. It should therefore be used only in specialist units where the staff are very experienced in its use and in monitoring its effects.

Ciclosporin offers great benefits to people who respond to it and who can avoid its side effects. Between 53 and 62 per cent of people with very severe ulcerative colitis who were given it in controlled trials had avoided surgery to remove the colon (colectomy) over the next 3 to 5 years of follow-up.[2] Experts recommend adding one of two other immunosuppressive drugs, azathioprine or 6-mercaptopurine, to ciclosporin as a further help in avoiding the need for colectomy.

Other treatments that have been tried include a variety of antibiotics, but the evidence that they help is sparse, and the researchers' attention has now focussed, as with Crohn's disease, on probiotics (see Chapter Six).

The probiotics used so far in ulcerative colitis (as opposed to Crohn's) include special strains of E. coli and combinations of bifidobacteria, lactobacilli and one-third harmless bacterium, *Streptococcus thermophilus*. The aim is to encourage an environment in the colon that will be beneficial to the mucosal cells, allowing them to heal and to build up their own immunity against possible pathogens. The presence of these probiotic bacteria in the colon will also act as powerful competitors to the growth of bacteria that might stimulate inflammation.

So far, probiotics have produced excellent results in a condition called 'pouchitis', which is ulcerative colitis in a 'pouch' of gut that has been left after colectomy. The need for a pouch is explained in the chapter on surgery.

Other approaches have included fish oil capsules and nicotine patches. The active ingredient of fish oil is 'eicosapentaenoic acid', which blocks excess immune reactivity. It has been reported as effective in mild to moderate ulcerative colitis, but patients had to take too many capsules a day. Many stopped taking the drug because it left a fishy smell on their breath. Mesalazine is just as effective, and does not pose the same problems.

Nicotine patches (remember that smokers have less ulcerative colitis than non-smokers) have also been tried. They do seem initially to control mild to moderate ulcerative colitis, but no more effectively than steroids, and they do not prolong the period between relapses. Nicotine enemas and delayed-release tablets are also in early trials.

Other proposed medications that need much further investigation before they can be used generally in ulcerative colitis include *Plantago ovata* seeds and the anticoagulant heparin. The first are digested by bacteria in the colon to produce a fatty acid called butyrate that is thought to be essential for the health of the colon mucosa cells. One theory is that the ulcers occur because the mucosa is starved of butyrate, so the seeds should remedy that deficiency. Very preliminary trials suggest that they may be as effective in maintaining a remission as mesalazine.[3]

Why heparin should be used is more difficult to understand. In theory, using an anticoagulant (that would prevent blood clotting) in a condition in which the gut is already bleeding should cause even more bleeding. However, it has other effects on cytokines which should damp down the inflammation and help the mucosal cells to heal. Current trial results are equivocal. An initial study suggested that it brought 75 per cent of patients with acute ulcerative colitis into remission, but follow-up studies have not been so definite in its favour. The jury is still out on heparin.

Finally, we can turn to infliximab. Its use in Crohn's has been described in Chapter Six. Infliximab is more appropriate to Crohn's, in theory, than to ulcerative colitis, because its target, TNF-α, plays a bigger part in causing Crohn's than ulcerative colitis. Yet preliminary reports in small numbers of patients strongly suggest that it is at least as effective in bringing about a remission in ulcerative colitis as in Crohn's. One found that 16 out of 17 patients with severe ulcerative colitis responded to infliximab.[4]

Chapter Eleven

Ulcerative Colitis – The Need for Follow-up

Once the initial episode of ulcerative colitis has settled, what next? If you have had just one bout of it, even if it has been a relatively minor attack, you must attend for follow-up. And that follow-up is for the rest of your life. That's because you are at higher risk than normal of developing colon cancer in the years to come, and the aim of follow-up is make sure that, if it does show signs of starting, it can be treated or prevented in time to save your life.

So what exactly are the risks for you, and how do today's doctors ensure that you keep your personal risk of cancer to a minimum?

First, the risk is related to the extent of the disease in your colon. The more surface area of your colon is affected, the higher is your risk of cancer. It is also related to the duration of your disease. The longer you have had ulcerative colitis, the higher is your cancer risk. Interestingly, the severity of the disease (that is its activity, as opposed to its area) does not seem to matter where cancer risk is concerned. Even disease that is in remission and not causing symptoms may increase the risk. The most reliable figures for risk in a large population were reported by A Ekbom and colleagues in 1990 in the *New England Journal of Medicine*.[1]

They calculated the risk to be 1.7 for patients with proctitis only (affecting only the rectum). This figure means that the rate of colon cancer in these patients was 1.7 times higher than that of the general population. The corresponding figures for people with colitis beyond the rectum as far as the transverse colon was 2.8. For those with disease extending into the ascending colon it was 14.8.

Other aspects of ulcerative colitis that increase the risk of cancer include having relatives with cancer of the colon or rectum, and involvement of the bile duct (a rare complication called primary sclerosing cholangitis). Spread of the ulceration back from the colon into the terminal ileum (the final part of the small intestine) also adds to the cancer risk.

The good news is that maintenance treatment with mesalazine and other aminosalicylates, cigarette smoking and possibly vitamin E and folic acid may protect against cancer. This must be the only beneficial action of cigarettes! (I must repeat here that nicotine patches may be a better choice, as cigarettes have so many other bad effects.)

If cancer does arise, it can start anywhere in the colon, and even appear at more than one site at a time, so it is essential to be seen regularly for a check. There are guidelines for specialists on how to perform the checks, but Richard Farrell and Mark Peppercorn of Harvard Medical School, writing in the *Lancet*,[2] state with concern that only a minority of British gastroenterologists follow them to the letter. So here is the ideal, according to doctors Farrell and Peppercorn.

Crucial to discovering the change from normal tissue to cancer is the discovery of 'dysplasia' (a specific change in the structure of cells) on microscope study of biopsies taken from colon mucosa. This is done under endoscopy, and is not particularly uncomfortable. The first problem for doctors Farrell and Peppercorn is that pathologists may fail to agree on what is and what isn't dysplasia leading to cancer.

The guidelines state, too, that people who have had ulcerative colitis extending to the middle and right side of the colon for seven years or more should be seen regularly. Those who have only had colitis in the left (descending) colon can wait until they have had it for 15 years before entering the surveillance programme. If they have had sclerosing cholangitis (see earlier paragraph), the screening starts without delay, after diagnosis.

Once a patient is in the programme, at each visit the endoscope is passed all the way to the caecum (the beginning of the colon). On the way at least 33 large biopsies are taken for scrutiny for dysplasia.

If the biopsies show no dysplasia at any site, the next visit is scheduled for between one and two years. If the biopsies show 'indefinite dysplasia', the inflammation is treated and the patient is seen in six months. If the mucosa looks flat on endoscopy and the biopsy taken from the site is dysplastic, two pathologists must discuss the slide and conclude that it is either high or low grade. If it is high grade, then the patient should have a colectomy. If low, then it can be postponed for six months and seen again.

The gastroenterologist may also see 'DALMs' while on the trip through your colon. These are Dysplasia-Associated Lesions or

Masses that look suspiciously like cancer to the experienced eye. If there is any suspicion that they are cancerous under the microscope, then colectomy is the only choice. Some DALMs turn out to be benign polyps, and not dysplastic or cancerous. In these cases, they can be removed under the endoscope and the colon can be preserved, at least for the time being. The patient must be seen again in a year.

Colectomy sounds a fearsome operation, but there are times when it is inevitable if you wish to survive. One of these is fulminating ulcerative colitis, when the bowel wall is deteriorating and peritonitis and septicaemia are imminent. The other, done under less frightening conditions, is colectomy for early cancer. They are described in Chapter Twelve.

Chapter Twelve

Surgery for Colitis

I first met patients with ulcerative colitis in a specialist ward as a medical student under Brian Brooke, at the Queen Elizabeth Hospital, Birmingham. The experience established my feelings about the severity of the disease and how it damaged people's quality of life. It wasn't until years later, in general practice, that I understood that there were people with inflammatory bowel disease who did not need surgery and who managed more or less happily to cope with it on medication alone.

Brian Brooke's patients had no choice. For them it was surgery or die. In his hands, of course, they did exceptionally well. It wasn't for us as his student 'dressers' to question how well they enjoyed life afterwards. They came into the ward very ill and left it very much better, and that was all that mattered.

In those days, Mr Brooke did one operation, a pan-proctocolectomy. He removed the whole of the colon and rectum, leaving the patient with an ileostomy in the lower right side of the abdomen. This was the terminal ileum, discharging its contents into a bag stuck to the abdominal wall. Professor Brooke devised the 'stoma', the opening of the ileum on the skin, so that it could be easily managed by the patient and was watertight. However, it was a source of permanent incontinence, and although the patients who had it were grateful still to be alive, they would very much have preferred to have been left with a way of emptying their bowel under their own control.

Today, pan-proctocolectomies are still done for people who need to be cured in one fell swoop and are not anxious about having to use an ileostomy bag. It is used, too, for older, frail people and for those with poor anal control, for whom saving the anus would still not prevent leakage, discomfort and embarrassment.

For the vast majority of patients with ulcerative colitis who need surgery, however, there are now better choices. The first of these is 'colectomy with ileorectostomy'. The colon is removed, but the rectum is preserved, and the terminal ileum is joined on to it. The anus and continence are preserved and the patient does not have an ileostomy.

At first sight, this appears vastly preferable to the Brooke pan-proctocolectomy, but it has two serious drawbacks. The first is that it does not cure the rectal disease, so that in some people leaving the rectum continues to give them discomfort. Worse, the rectum may become affected by a stricture (narrowing) due to scarring or active disease. That can lead to a lot of discomfort and either considerable difficulty in defecation or incontinence. The other drawback is that the rectum retains the extra risk of becoming cancerous. The patient has to return every year or so to be examined and for biopsies to be taken to detect dysplasia (see Chapter Eleven). One in ten patients who have had ileorectostomies eventually have to have their rectum removed because of suspicious changes or frank cancer. Because of this, colectomy with ileorectostomies are now usually restricted to older patients (the over-sixties) for whom the subsequent cancer risk is relatively low.

The third option is a proctocolectomy with Kock's continent ileostomy. There is no need here to go into details of how Kock's ileostomy is fashioned. It is enough to know that just under the stoma the end of the ileum is fashioned into a pouch with what is best described as a 'nipple' valve at its end. The stoma is flush with the wall of the abdomen, instead of protruding like the Brooke ileostomy, and it can be placed low down on near the right groin so that it is unobtrusive. It is emptied by passing a small tube, quite painlessly, into the pouch and emptying the contents directly into a toilet. There is no need for bags. The stoma can be hidden by a bikini, so that young women can wear swimsuits without embarrassment. All it needs is a small piece of gauze on the surface of the stoma to take up the small amount of mucus that oozes from the exposed circle of ileum.

Occasionally people who have been given a pouch suddenly develop a watery, often blood-stained diarrhoea, with stomach cramps and a mild temperature rise. This is 'pouchitis' and is caused by a bacterial infection. Happily it almost always responds very well to the antimicrobial drug metronidazole: it is very rare for pouchitis to be so bad that the stoma needs another operation and the pouch to be replaced.

The Kock pouch operation is often offered to people with Brooke operations who want a more comfortable life and to get rid of their bag. It is also used for people for whom an ileo-anal anastomosis (junction) is not feasible or has failed.

The fourth choice is the Rolls-Royce of ulcerative colitis surgery. It is proctocolectomy with ileal pouch-anal anastomosis. It is not yet perfected, but when it is successful it leaves a better quality of life than the other three options. The surgeon removes the whole colon and the upper rectum, and then removes the mucosa from the lower rectum, thereby removing the risk of future cancer. An ileal pouch is then joined to the upper part of the anus. That allows for a good faecal reservoir, similar to that of the sigmoid colon, and preserves the ability to defecate voluntarily. There is no stoma. This type of surgery avoids damaging the nerves to the bladder and to the penis in men, so that there is little risk of the incontinence or impotence that sometimes dogged the patient after the older Brooke operation. It also relieves the patient of having to wait for the wound to heal where the anus has been – often a real problem after the other operations.

Anyone going in for ulcerative colitis surgery should discuss the options with the surgeon. If at all possible, ileal pouch-anal anastomosis should be the operation of choice.

What can you expect in the long term after ileal pouch-anal anastomosis? I have in front of me as I write a rsum of the first 670 patients given this operation at the Mayo clinic.[1] They were treated more than ten years ago, so presumably the Mayo team will have even better results now, as they have gained experience.

After follow-up for between six months and eight years, every patient could manage to open their 'neorectum' (as the authors call it) spontaneously. They passed five stools a day and one at night. Eighty-three per cent had no daytime incontinence and 56 per cent had perfect night-time continence. Forty per cent had occasional night-time spotting. Eight per cent had some sexual dysfunction, including impotence and ejaculation problems in the men and painful intercourse in the women. Twenty-two per cent (148 of the 670 patients) had had pouchitis, but in every case it had settled on metronidazole taken by mouth. Forty-eight patients (6 per cent) had to have further operations because of infections in the pelvis, or because they turned out to have Crohn's disease, or because their neorectum had not worked well enough.

These are good results, but of course not perfect. They would probably have been better still if more patients had been sent for surgery sooner: many were quite ill because their surgery had been delayed. It would be interesting to see how the 1991 results compare with today's, and how the Mayo Clinic results compare with those of the average British hospital.

Chapter Thirteen

Surgery for Crohn's Disease

Surgery is always a treatment of last resort for Crohn's disease. That's because it is usually widespread throughout the small intestine, so that it is impossible in many cases to remove all the diseased gut. If that were attempted, it might leave the patient with too little remaining gut, which would reduce very considerably his or her ability to digest food. More than that, surgery for Crohn's disease has the unfortunate, and sometimes tragic, effect of sometimes leaving the patient with fistulas, either to the skin or between loops of gut, that are impossible to heal. These can leave people with a permanent discharging hole in the skin of the abdomen, or permanent and copious diarrhoea. This is quite unlike the case for surgery in ulcerative colitis, which is confined to obvious sites in the colon, which can easily be defined and removed. After surgery for ulcerative colitis, fistulas do not form and the patient improves in health and quality of life, sometimes immeasurably so.

However, there are times when surgery is essential for people with Crohn's. Very rarely, patches of Crohn's in the small intestine develop a hole ('perforation') that leads from the lumen into the peritoneal cavity around it. This leads to peritonitis, and emergency surgery is needed to save the patient's life. That involves removing the segment of bowel that contains the perforation, tying off the gut beyond it so that it does not leak, and bringing the end of the gut above it to the surface in a temporary ileostomy. After the surgery, and having waited for a time (usually several weeks) for the gut to heal, the ileostomy is put back and re-joined with the lower bowel, so that normal life can be resumed. In the meantime, the main priority for the patient is to keep well nourished. Sometimes a formula diet is needed.

In Crohn's colitis, the inflammation spreads through the ileo-caecal valve into the colon. There the disease can become as acute as fulminant ulcerative colitis (see Chapter Nine), with severe bleeding. The rule of thumb operated by most specialist units is that, if more than four units of blood are being lost in each 24 hours, surgery is needed. For Crohn's colitis, this means a proctocolectomy with ileostomy similar to the surgery described in the previous chapter for ulcerative colitis. An advantage for the Crohn's patient is that the rectum can be left in place to allow the patient to have the end of the ileum joined with the rectum, and to have complete control over their bowel movements.

The most serious complication of Crohn's is 'toxic megacolon', in which the colon becomes highly inflamed, leading to bleeding and perforation, with peritonitis, septicaemia and death within a few days if it is not treated correctly. According to Professor B G Wolff of the Mayo Clinic, toxic megacolon affects one in five of his patients with Crohn's. This seems to me to be very high: I wonder if his patients generally have more severe Crohn's than those seen by less eminent doctors.

Whether or not it is as common as Professor Wolff says, toxic megacolon must be operated upon very quickly to save the patient's life. The standard operation is proctocolectomy, saving the rectum where possible for future link-up with the ileum. Sometimes part of the colon can be preserved: this allows the patient to pass fewer stools per day after recovery. Medical treatment alone fails to save around one-third of people with it, and of those who survive around one in five have another episode of toxic megacolon. Patients undergoing surgery for it need to have antibiotic cover before, during and after the operation.

Some patients with Crohn's can benefit from 'elective' surgery. This is surgery done in a non-emergency setting for particular complications. The most common is to relieve a stricture – a narrowed segment of small bowel that is obstructing the normal flow of bowel contents. The surgeon doesn't necessarily have to cut out the stricture. He may manage to open out the section of bowel with a 'stricturoplasty', in which the wall of the narrowed piece of bowel is opened lengthwise and then stitched 'acrosswise'. The resultant segment of bowel is slightly shorter than before, but much wider and the contents can pass through it. The operation avoids cutting out a segment of the bowel, minimizing the possibility of spread of the disease along the junction line. Other reasons for elective surgery include the removal of a fistula between two loops of gut, or to remove a section of gut, bleeding from which has caused severe anaemia. The problem with both of these operations is that they tend to leave further complications, such as adhesions (loops of bowel stuck together) or even more fistulas, in their wake.

As more effective medical treatments for Crohn's have evolved, the numbers of people with Crohn's who need surgery are falling. Ideally, the aim is to avoid surgery altogether, but that will not happen in the foreseeable future.

Chapter Fourteen

Irritable Bowel and Coeliac Disease

Neither irritable bowel nor coeliac disease can strictly be called examples of colitis, but they are included in this book because their symptoms can be so similar to those of Crohn's and ulcerative colitis.

Irritable Bowel

I have had a long and not entirely successful relationship with irritable bowel. Here I must refer again to Brian Brooke. In his 1986 textbook, *The Troubled Gut*, he devotes only two pages to irritable bowel. He describes it as a 'strange equivocal condition seen all too often in gastrointestinal clinics throughout the world'. I remember Professor Brooke's frustration at the patients with irritable bowel who came to him believing they had something worse. He was often the second or third consultant they had visited because they would not believe the opinions of lesser, more mortal, physicians. He saw irritable bowel sufferers as wasting his time, when he wanted to get on with treating people whom he saw as having 'real' problems – his colitis patients.

In a way, he was right. He writes that 'The best treatment for irritable bowel lies with the doctor who is prepared to listen, who is able to recognize the condition from the story, who has the strength of mind to avoid recourse to investigation, and last but not least who will spend as much time as is needed to explain the situation. It is remarkable how the symptoms ease to tolerable proportions, if not totally, when suspicion and fear are properly allayed.'

His clinic was not one in which the doctor could spend the time needed to help patients with irritable bowel.

My views on irritable bowel as a young general practitioner were modelled on Professor Brooke's. Whenever people came to me with new symptoms that might be due to irritable bowel, I tried to take time to talk to them about the illness, and to avoid, whenever I could, sending them for investigations. That wasn't easy because we had no clear, proven treatment for irritable bowel, and the patients naturally kept coming back. The fact that I could do little for them made them think the diagnosis was being missed. The result? In the end, most of them did make the journey up to hospital to see our gastroenterologists, who soon made the same diagnosis and sent them back to me, no better and little the wiser.

After six years in general practice, I decided on a career change, and entered medical research. One of my first jobs was to help to develop, by planning and overseeing clinical trials, the first drug specifically designed to help irritable bowel. This was mebeverine, otherwise known as Colofac.

It wasn't long before I came up against an almost insoluble problem. How could I measure the intensity of episodes of irritable bowel in such a way as to be able to analyse the results mathematically? We had to find a way of putting numbers on symptoms and signs, and then measuring the difference after treatment with the drug or placebo. Irritable bowel symptoms are not easily enumerated. The main ones are abdominal discomfort, bloating and changes in the pattern and number of the bowel movements. The problem was that sometimes the same type of bowel movements were described by two different patients in two different ways. What would you call the passing of a shower of small hard pellets like rabbit droppings? We found some people who would call it constipation, and others who were sure it was diarrhoea. As for putting numbers on discomfort in the abdomen, or the need to strain to pass a motion, our statistician would quietly sit in a corner and weep.

I was fortunate in having Dr John Cumming, doctor to the students at Reading University, as a colleague. John, sadly, died too young, but one instrument he left to posterity was his 'fartometer'. This was a microphone that was fixed to a belt that was strapped round the patient's midriff. The patient wore it for 24 hours, and recorded the sounds made by his gut throughout that time. We were left with hours of tapes, recording gurgles, rumbles and other sounds less easy to describe in a respectable book.

The idea of the fartometer was brilliant. We thought at the time that the more active a bowel was, the louder and more frequent would be the sounds we collected. The less active the bowel, the quieter the abdomen. We were confident that differences in the sound loudness, quality or frequency would in some way relate to the symptoms of irritable bowel, although at that time we didn't know whether irritable bowel was the result of an over- or under-active bowel.

What we actually found was a complete surprise. The fartometer was used in hundreds of subjects, some with and some without irritable bowel. Absolutely nothing we heard bore any relationship to the symptoms of the disease. If the sounds that emanated from the abdomen were any indication of the activity of the bowel, then the symptoms of irritable bowel did not co-ordinate with them. Irritable bowel was not a result of either an under-active or an over-active bowel. The symptoms could occur when it was quiet or extremely noisy. And we could find no general difference in the bowel sound pattern between irritable bowel sufferers and those who had never had symptoms of the illness.

Where did that leave us? In the first place, without results to publish – so you are reading the outcome of that research for the first time in this book. But it meant that if we were to find what causes the symptoms of irritable bowel, we had to use more sophisticated and scientific systems to measure them. The next step was to use an electronic 'pill' that measured pressures around it and sent the results out by radio signals. The subject of the research swallowed the pill, which could then be followed on its travel through the body, repeatedly measuring the pressures around it in the stomach, small intestine and colon. Finally it was excreted, picked up and washed (thoroughly!) and used again by the next patient. Honestly, these people did give their fully informed consent to the studies. Nowadays the pills are only used once and then discarded.

The pressure studies didn't help much either. There was no convincing link between pressure inside the bowel and symptoms of irritable colon – the irritable colon sufferers showed the same patterns and the same timing of passage from mouth to anus as the volunteers without symptoms. We still did not have the concrete measurements we needed to perform proper statistical analysis on the benefits and drawbacks of our proposed treatment.

Eventually we had to rely on asking patients to write down their impressions of the severity and timing of their symptoms, and we tried to analyse the differences between the days on drug and days on placebo. The results were still unsatisfactory, as it was very difficult for patients to make this assessment reliably from day to day.

So why was this research so difficult, when the condition is so common in every developed country? International committees have struggled for years to find ways of diagnosing irritable bowel reliably, while ruling out more serious disease like Crohn's and ulcerative colitis, and even cancer of the bowel and coeliac diseases. In 1999 this came to fruition when a working party from Europe and North America designed the ROME II criteria for making the diagnosis of irritable bowel.[1]

ROME II defines irritable bowel as follows:

The patient has had, for 12 weeks, which need not be consecutive, in the previous 12 months, abdominal discomfort or pain with two of the following three features:

- relief on defecation
- onset linked to a change in the frequency of stools
- onset linked with a change in the appearance of the stool

Symptoms that support the diagnosis include:

- fewer than three motions per week
- more than three motions per day
- hard or lumpy stools
- loose or watery stools
- need to strain to open the bowel
- the feeling of urgency (to have to rush to get to the toilet) to open the bowel
- the feeling afterwards that the bowel movement was not complete
- the passing of mucus (white, phlegm-like material) during a bowel movement
- a bloated, swollen, full-feeling abdomen
- Symptoms against the diagnosis of irritable bowel, and which should mean further investigations, include:
- weight loss
- bleeding along with the diarrhoea
- diarrhoea at night that disturbs sleep
- anaemia

Looking at these criteria for irritable bowel diagnosis, it is not surprising that British general practitioners have estimated that around 15 per cent of the population have it. What ROME II is describing is how the bowel reacts the next day to the previous heavy night out. And for many others, these symptoms may just be the bowel 'complaining' at a diet of fast food or too much to eat, too little of which is fruit, vegetable and fibre.

If you recognize your symptoms in this list, then you almost certainly have irritable bowel and not colitis. You do not need further investigations. But you may need a lot of advice about what and how much you eat and drink, and how much you exercise. You may also need advice on how to cope with stress, because anxiety and depression both seem to be linked to irritable bowel symptoms, perhaps by giving us a heightened awareness of our inner workings. When we worry or are under stress, we feel our heart beating faster, our mouth and throat becoming drier, and our neck muscles tensing. Becoming aware of our insides churning is part of the same mechanism.

Some investigators, indeed, believe that irritable bowel is merely the patient becoming aware of his or her insides. Once you do become aware of your bowel making noises, it can become difficult to ignore it. I'm not sure I buy that message in its entirety. There may be some truth in it, but there is also no doubt that irritable bowel is a physical entity, and that it can be helped by drugs as well as lifestyle advice.

The current drugs that are licensed for use in irritable bowel in Britain still include mebeverine, my drug project from so many years ago. I'm pleased about that because it means that the drug was of use, despite all our fruitless efforts to prove that it worked. It acts directly on the bowel wall muscle, relieving cramp. Similar direct-acting antispasmodics are alverine and colpermine, this last being peppermint oil. Antispasmodics are mainly prescribed for people whose symptoms are mostly abdominal spasms, cramps and pain, or frequent bouts of diarrhoea. Laxatives such as lactulose (that do not cause the muscle of the bowel wall to constrict) are usually the drug of first choice for people whose main symptom is constipation. It goes without saying, however, that everyone with irritable bowel should look at their lifestyle, and not just depend on a prescription alone.

If you have irritable bowel, what you eat matters. The trouble is that for different people it matters in different ways. Some people need more fruit and fibre and less meat and dairy products to feel better. Others feel worse when they fill their colon with such residue, and feel better on a lighter diet that gives them a smaller stool. You will not know which type you are until you try both. Then it is up to you to be disciplined enough to keep to the eating habit that suits you most.

Coeliac Disease

The last paragraph about irritable bowel and eating habits is the perfect entry to the section on coeliac disease because if there is one cause of diarrhoea that depends absolutely on what you eat – or more specifically what you don't eat – it is coeliac disease. That was proved beyond doubt in 1945, when the retreating Nazis decided to starve the Dutch by taking almost all of the food grown in the Netherlands back to Germany. The whole Dutch population suffered terribly. Many were starving when the war finished in May.

Yet one group of children did remarkably well. Without bread or food made from flour, they suddenly began to grow and feel much healthier. They were the children with an illness the cause of which was unknown, but was named coeliac disease. Children affected by it failed to grow, were thin and listless, and had daily diarrhoea. The diarrhoea was full of fat and was very unpleasant for the children. Few of them grew to maturity, most dying of malnutrition in their later childhood.

The doctors looking after them in 1945 were staggered by their seemingly miraculous recovery when deprived of bread. Luckily they came to the right conclusion and continued the ban on bread and wheat flour even after the end of the war, when they were again in plentiful supply. Soon after that, it became clear that children with coeliac disease were reacting badly to gluten, an ingredient of wheat flour, and of some other cereals. The usual healthy columns and crypts of their small intestinal mucosa were replaced by a thin, flat layer of cells that were obviously unhealthy and unable to digest food residues properly and efficiently. When all gluten was excluded from their food, the small bowel soon recovered and the columns and crypts returned. The mucosal cells looked normal and functioned perfectly, and normal digestion resumed. Children whose previous outlook had been grim could now look forward to a healthy and long life, provided they stayed off gluten.

Today doctors are extremely well aware that children who are not thriving should be tested for coeliac disease. Few children with diarrhoea escape the net. Happily, they don't need to undergo endoscopy to make the diagnosis. People with coeliac disease carry in their blood substances called endomysial antibodies, or EMA. These can be identified by a standard blood test. Once EMA has been found in your blood, you can start on your gluten-free future, and feel better after only a day or two. Children with coeliac disease, once they stop eating gluten, grow like mushrooms (which, of course, are gluten-free).

So why is coeliac disease featured in a book on colitis? In the last few years we have come to recognize that some adults with diarrhoea have a form of coeliac disease that did not affect them in childhood. Their symptoms could be confused with irritable bowel syndrome.

In November 2001, David Sanders and his colleagues of the Royal Hallamshire Hospital, Sheffield reported on blood antibody tests in 300 patients consecutively attending their university clinic with all the symptoms of irritable bowel according to the ROME II criteria.[2] They compared them with 300 similar 'control' subjects without irritable bowel symptoms. Fourteen of the 300 patients, and two of the 300 controls, turned out to have adult coeliac disease. Eleven of the patients and both of the controls were positive for EMA. The three patients who had negative EMA results had 'antigliadin' antibodies, another test that helps to confirm coeliac disease.

Dr Sanders' group advised from these results that people thought to have irritable bowel syndrome should have at least one investigation – an EMA test to rule out coeliac disease. Antigliadin tests may also be useful. They added that trying to diagnose adult coeliac disease from the symptoms was not so helpful. They found coeliac disease in two of 62 irritable bowel patients in whom constipation dominated, in four of 84 with mainly diarrhoea, and in eight of 154 patients in whom diarrhoea and constipation alternated.

Their report started a debate among the Lancet's experts. One, Roland Valori of the Gloucestershire Hospital, wrote that he was screening for coeliac disease more and more patients with a wide range of odd bowel symptoms that do not fit neatly into the ROME

II criteria. He added that 'very few of my patients with unexplained gastroenterological symptoms fit neatly into the ROME II criteria'. For him, 'selecting patients for investigations for coeliac disease will continue to depend on subtle factors that are not so easily measured by a set of diagnostic factors'.

What is the message from this chapter? That, in general, if you have repeated symptoms which fit with irritable bowel syndrome, then you don't need to be investigated for every possible eventuality. You can believe your doctor and consultant if they are happy that there is nothing more than irritable bowel. However, it would be worth asking them if they have excluded adult coeliac disease. Blood tests to check on antigliadins (gliadin is a constituent of gluten) are one way, such as the EMA test mentioned above.

It is important that the diagnosis is either made or ruled out, because adult coeliac disease is just as eminently treatable as the childhood form. It responds extremely well and fast to exclusion of gluten from your food. People with adult coeliac disease usually have symptoms which suggest that they are not fully digesting their food. They have diarrhoea and a bloated abdomen, yet lose weight and become anaemic and show signs of vitamin deficiency. These are all reversed by gluten exclusion.

However, we are increasingly recognizing that there is a less typical, or 'silent', form of adult coeliac disease. They may have no bowel problems. Instead they complain of tiredness, and tests show they have anaemia, osteoporosis, difficulty in walking ('ataxia') or peripheral neuropathy. People with peripheral neuropathy complain of numbness, pins and needles, and weakness in their limbs. They may also find problems knowing where their feet are in space (loss of 'position sense') and may lose their sense of detection of heat and cold. Amazingly, all these symptoms, which are related to lack of digestion of vitamins, disappear by simply avoiding gluten.

The 14 patients described by Dr Sanders probably fell into a group of people midway between the 'typical' and 'silent' adult coeliacs. They had a few bowel symptoms, but not enough to classify them as 'typical' and too many to be 'silent' cases. Doctors like myself will have to look out for them in future among our mass of people diagnosed with irritable bowel. And people with irritable bowel should know about it themselves, so that they can ask the right questions. Let us hope they always get the correct answers.

Appendix

Why You Mustn't Smoke – And How to Stop If You Do

Smoking is a stupid, suicidal habit for anyone, no matter how healthy. It is even worse, if that is possible, for people with Crohn's because it is implicated in causing the disease, and makes the inflammation in the bowel worse. That is on top of the extra risks of heart disease, stroke, lung disease and kidney disease faced by all smokers. So if you are a smoker, you must be a non-smoker before you put this book down.

How Smoking Harms You

Tobacco smoke contains carbon monoxide and nicotine. The first poisons the red blood cells, so that they cannot pick up and distribute much-needed oxygen to the organs and tissues, including the heart muscle. Carbon monoxide-affected red cells (in the 20-a-day smoker, nearly 20 per cent of red cells are carrying carbon monoxide instead of oxygen) are also stiffer than normal, so that they can't bend and flex through the smallest blood vessels. The gas also directly poisons the heart muscle, so that it cannot contract properly and efficiently, thereby delivering a 'double whammy' of damage.

Nicotine causes small arteries to narrow, so that the blood flow through them slows. It raises blood cholesterol levels, thickening the blood and promoting the degenerative process in the endothelium of the small arteries. Both nicotine and carbon monoxide encourage the blood to clot, multiplying the risks of coronary thrombosis and a thrombotic stroke even more.

Add to all this the tars that smoke deposits in the lungs, which further reduce the ability of red cells to pick up oxygen, and the scars and damage to the endothelium in the lungs that always lead to chronic bronchitis and often to cancer, and you have a formula for disaster.

The Bald Facts

If these facts about smoking do not convince you to stop, then you may as well not have read this book, because there is no point in being 'health conscious' if you continue to indulge in tobacco. Its ill-effects will counterbalance any good that your doctors or other lifestyle changes and medication can do for you.

- Smokers have a much higher risk of developing Crohn's than non-smokers. If they continue to smoke, their disease is much more severe than in those who stop.
- Smoking causes more deaths from heart attacks than from lung cancer or bronchitis.
- People who smoke have two or three times the risk of a fatal heart attack that non-smokers have. The risk rises with the number of cigarettes smoked per day.
- Men under 45 who smoke 25 or more cigarettes a day have a 10 to 15 times greater chance of death from a heart attack than non-smoking men of the same age.
- About 40 per cent of all heavy smokers die before they reach 65. Of those who reach that age, many are disabled by bronchitis, angina, heart failure and leg amputations, all because they smoke. A high cholesterol and/or triglyceride level makes all these risks of smoking much greater. Only 10 per cent of smokers survive in reasonable health to age 75. Most non-smokers reach 75 in good health.
- In Britain, 40 per cent of all cancer deaths are from lung cancer, which is very rare in non-smokers. Of 441 British male doctors who died from lung cancer, only seven had never smoked. Only one non-smoker in 60 develops lung cancer: the figure for heavy smokers is one in six!
- Other cancers more common in smokers than in non-smokers include tongue, throat, larynx, pancreas, kidney, bladder and cervical cancers.
- No More Excuses

The very fact that you are reading this book means that you are taking an intelligent interest in your health. So, after reading so far, it should be common sense to you not to smoke. Yet it is very difficult to stop, and many people who need an excuse for not stopping put up spurious arguments for their stance. Here are ones that every doctor is tired of hearing, and my replies:

My father/grandfather smoked 20 a day and lived till he was 75.
Everyone knows someone like that, but they conveniently forget the many others they have known who died long before their time. The chances are that you will be one of them, rather than one of the lucky few.

People who don't smoke also have heart attacks.
True. There are other causes of heart attacks, but 70 per cent of all people under 65 admitted to coronary care with heart attacks are smokers, as are 91 per cent of people with angina considered for coronary bypass surgery.

I believe in moderation in all things, and I only smoke moderately.
That's rubbish. We don't accept moderation in mugging, or dangerous driving, or exposure to asbestos (which, incidentally, causes far fewer deaths from lung cancer than smoking). Younger men who are only moderate smokers have a much higher risk of heart attack than non-smoking men of the same age.

I can cut down on cigarettes, but I can't stop.
It won't do you much good if you do. People who cut down usually inhale more from each cigarette and leave a smaller butt, so that they end up with the same blood levels of nicotine and carbon monoxide. You must stop completely.

I'm just as likely to be run over in the road as to die from my smoking.
In Britain about 15 people die on the roads each day. This contrasts with 100 deaths a day from lung cancer, 100 from chronic bronchitis and 100 from heart attacks, almost all of which are due to smoking. Of every 1,000 young men who smoke, on average one will be murdered, six will die on the roads, and 250 will die from their smoking habit.

I have to die of something.
In my experience this is always said by someone in good health. They

no longer say it after their heart attack or stroke, or after they have coughed up blood.

I don't want to be old, anyway.
We define 'old' differently as we grow older. Most of us would like to live a long time, without the inconvenience of being old. If we take care of ourselves on the way to becoming old, we have at least laid the foundations for enjoying our old age.

I'd rather die of a heart attack than something else.
Most of us would like a quick death, but many heart attack victims leave a grieving partner in their early 50s to face 30 years of loneliness. Is that really what you wish?

Stress, not smoking, is the main cause of heart attacks.
Not true. Stress is very difficult to measure, and very difficult to relate to heart attack rates. In any case, you have to cope with stress whether you smoke or not. Smoking is an extra burden that can never help, and it does not relieve stress. It isn't burning the candle at both ends that causes harm, but burning the cigarette at one end.

I'll stop when I start to feel ill.
That would be fine if the first sign of illness were not a full-blown heart attack from which more than a third die in the first four hours. It's too late to stop then.

I'll put on weight if I stop smoking.
You probably will, because your appetite will return and you will be able to taste food again. But the benefits of stopping smoking far outweigh the few extra pounds you may put on.

I enjoy smoking and don't want to give it up.
Is that really true? Is that not just an excuse because you can't stop? Ask yourself what your real pleasure is in smoking, and try to be honest with your answer.

Cigarettes settle my nerves. If I stopped I'd have to take a tranquillizer.
Smoking is a prop, like a baby's dummy, but it solves nothing. It doesn't remove any causes of stress, and only makes things worse

because it adds a promoter of bad health. And when you start to have symptoms, like the regular morning cough, it only makes you worry more.

I'll change to a pipe or cigar – they are safer.
Lifelong pipe and cigar smokers are less prone than cigarette smokers to heart attacks, but have five times the risk of lung cancer and ten times the risk of chronic bronchitis that non-smokers have. Cigarette smokers who switch to pipes or cigars continue to be at high risk of heart attack, probably because they inhale.

I've been smoking for 30 years – it's too late to stop now.
It's not too late whenever you stop. The risk of sudden death from a first heart attack falls away very quickly after stopping, even after a lifetime of smoking. If you stop after surviving a heart attack then you halve the risk of a second. It takes longer to reduce your risk of lung cancer, but it falls by 80 per cent over the next 15 years, no matter how long you have been a smoker.

I wish I could stop. I've tried everything, but nothing has worked.
Stopping smoking isn't easy unless you really want to do it. You have to make the effort yourself, rather than think that someone else can do it for you. So you must be motivated. If the next few pages do not motivate you, then nothing will.

How to Stop Smoking

You must find the right reason for yourself to stop. For someone with Crohn's, one reason is that it will help to improve your general health and make your illness less severe. The statistics for men and women who smoke are frightening enough, but there are plenty of other reasons.

If you are a teenager or in your early twenties, who sees middle age and sickness as remote possibilities, and smoking as exciting and dangerous, the best motivation to stop may be to think of the way it makes you look and smell. You can also add the environmental pollution of cigarette ends, and the way big business exploits Third World nations, keeping their populations in poverty while they make huge profits putting land that should be growing food under tobacco cultivation. Pakistan uses 120,000 acres and Brazil half a million acres of their richest agricultural land to grow tobacco. As the multinationals are now promoting their product very heavily to the developing world, no young adult who smokes can claim to be really concerned about the health of the Third World. This may be more likely to persuade you to stop (or not to start) than any thought about your own health or looks.

Smoking ages people prematurely, causing wrinkles and giving a pale, pasty complexion. Women smokers experience the menopause at an earlier age, even in their mid-thirties, which can destroy the plans of businesswomen to have their families after they have established themselves in a career. Smoking plus a high triglyceride level, an extremely common combination in women, vastly increases your chances of having a heart attack or stroke. It removes all your natural advantages over men in your protection against heart attack.

Let us assume you are now fully motivated. How do you stop? It is easy. You become a non-smoker, as if you had never smoked. You throw away all your cigarettes, and decide never to buy or accept another one. Announce the fact to all your friends, who will usually support you, and that's that. Most people find that they don't have true withdrawal symptoms, provided they are happy to stop. A few become agitated, irritable, nervous and can't sleep at night. But people who have had to stop for medical reasons – say, because they have been admitted to coronary care – hardly ever have withdrawal symptoms. This strongly suggests that the withdrawal symptoms are psychological rather than physical.

If you can last a week or two without a smoke, you will probably never light up again. The desire to smoke will disappear as the levels of carbon monoxide, nicotine and tarry chemicals in your lungs, blood, brain and other organs gradually subside.

If you must stop gradually, plan ahead. Write down a diary of the cigarettes you will have, leaving out one or two each succeeding day, and stick to it. Carry nicotine chewing gum or get a patch if you must, but remember that the nicotine is still harmful. Don't look on it as a long-term alternative to a smoke.

If you are having real difficulty stopping, ask your doctor for a prescription of Zyban. You may be offered a two-month course of the drug. It helps, but is by no means infallible.

If you do use aids to stop (others include acupuncture and hypnosis), remember they have no magical properties. They are a crutch to lean on while you make the determined effort to stop altogether. They cannot help if your will to stop is weak.

Recognize, too, that stopping smoking is not an end in itself. It is only part of your new way of life, which includes a new way of eating and exercise, and your new attitude to your future health. And you owe it not only to yourself but also to your partner, children, family and friends, because it will help to give them a healthier you for, hopefully, years to come.

You are not on your own. More than a million Britons have stopped smoking each year for the last 15 years. Only 1 in 3 adults now smokes (fewer than 1 in 20 doctors). By stopping, you are joining the sensible majority.

References

ChapterThree
1.   *Lancet*, 21-28 December 2002:2052

Chapter Five
1.   Hellers, G, 'Crohn's disease in Stockholm county 1955-1974. A study of epidemiology, results of surgical treatment and long-term proposals', *Acta Chirurgica Scandinavia* supp. 490 (1979)
2.   Armitage, E, et al., 'Incidence of juvenile-onset Crohn's disease in Scotland'. *Lancet* 353 (1979): 1496-1497
3.   Farthing, M J G, *Inflammatory Bowel Disease* (Chapman & Hall Medical, 1992) p. 19

Chapter Six
1.   Hampe, J et al., 'Association between insertion mutation in NOD2 gene and Crohn's disease in German and British populations', *Lancet* 357 (2001): 1925-1928
2.   Professor Shanahan, *Lancet* 5 January 2002:65
3.   Blumberg, R S et al., 'Animal models of mucosal inflammation and their relation to human inflammatory bowel disease', *Current Opinion Immunology* 11 (1999): 648-656. Wirtz, S and Neurath, M F, 'Animal models of intestinal inflammation: new insights into the molecular pathogenesis and immunotherapy of inflammatory bowel disease', *International Journal of Colorectal Disease* 15 (2000): 144-160
4.   Shanahan, F, 'Probiotics and inflammatory bowel disease: is there a scientific rationale?', *Inflammatory Bowel Disease* 6 (2000): 107-115
5.   Dieckgraefe, B K and Korzenick, J R, 'Treatment of active Crohn's disease with recombinant human granulocyte-macrophage colony stimulating factor', *Lancet* 360 (2002): 1478-1480

Chapter Seven
1.   Warthin, T A, 'Some epidemiological observations on the aetiology of regional enteritis', *Transactions of the American Clinical and Climatological Association* 80 (1969): 116-124

2.Gilat,T et al.,'Childhood factors in ulcerative colitis and Crohn's disease. An international co-operative study', *Scandinavian Journal of Gastroenterology* 22 (1987): 1009-1024

3.Logan, R F A and Kay, C R, 'Oral contraception, smoking and inflammatory bowel disease: findings in the Royal College of General Practitioners Oral Contraceptive Study', *International Journal of Epidemiology* 18 (1989): 105-107. Vessey, M et al., 'Chronic inflammatory bowel disease, cigarette smoking and use of oral contraceptives: findings in a large cohort study of women of childbearing age', *British Medical Journal* 292 (1986): 1101-1103

4.Boyko, E J et al.,'Risk of ulcerative colitis amongst former smokers', *New England Journal of Medicine* 316 (1987): 707-710

5.Penny, W J et al., 'Prevalence of inflammatory bowel disease amongst Mormons in Britain and Ireland', *Social Science Medicine* 21 (1985): 287-290

6.Present, D et al., *New England Journal of Medicine* 340 (1999): 1398-1405

7.Weedon, D D et al.,'Crohn's disease and cancer', *New England Journal of Medicine* 289 (1973): 1099-1103

8.Prior, P et al.,'Mortality in Crohn's disease', *Gastroenterology* 80 (1981): 307-312

9.Hanauer, S B et al.,'Maintenance infliximab for Crohn's disease: the ACCENT I randomised trial', *Lancet* 359 (2002): 1541-1549

Chapter Eight

1.Kelly, S M et al.,'Food intolerance in Crohn's disease', in *Inflammatory Bowel Disease*, editors Anagnostides, A A et al. (Chapman & Hall Medical, London 1991) p. 316-328

2.Workman, E et al., 'Diet in the management of Crohn's disease', *Human Nutrition and Applied Nutrition* 384 (1984): 4

Chapter Nine

1.Andresen, A F R, 'Gastrointestinal manifestations of food allergy', *Medical Journal and Record* 122 (1925): 271-275

2.Truelove, S C, 'Ulcerative Colitis provoked by milk', *British Medical Journal* 1 (1962): 154-160

3.Mayberry, J F, 'Epidemiology of inflammatory bowel disease: a European perspective', in *Inflammatory Bowel Disease*, editors

Anagnostides, A A et al. (Chapman & Hall, London 1991) p. 172

4.Lindberg, E et al., 'Smoking and inflammatory bowel disease: a case control study', *Gut* 29 (1988): 352-357

5.Evans, J M et al., 'Non-steroidal anti-inflammatory drugs are associated with emergency admission to hospital for colitis due to inflammatory bowel disease', *Gut* 40 (1997): 619-622

6.Andersson, R E et al., 'Appendectomy and protection against ulcerative colitis', *New England Journal of Medicine* 344 (2001): 808-814

Chapter Ten

1.Lichtiger, S et al., 'Cyclosporine in severe ulcerative colitis refractory to steroid therapy', *New England Journal of Medicine* 330 (1994): 1841-1845. Van Gossum, A et al., 'Short and long term efficacy of cyclosporin administration in patients with acute severe ulcerative colitis: Belgian IBD group', *Acta Gastroenterologica Belgica* 60 (1997): 197-200. Carbonnel, F et al., 'Intravenous cyclosporine in attacks of ulcerative colitis: short term and long term responses', *Digest Disease Science* 41 (1996): 2471-2476

2.Stack, W A et al., 'Short term and long term outcome of patients treated with cyclosporin for severe acute ulcerative colitis', *Alimentary Pharmacological Therapy* 12 (1998): 973-978. Cohen, R D et al., 'Intravenous cyclosporin in ulcerative colitis: a five year experience', *American Journal of Gastroenterology* 94 (1999): 1587-1592

3.Fernandez-Benares, F et al., 'Randomized clinical trial of Plantago ovata seeds (dietary fibre) as compared with mesalamine in maintaining remission in ulcerative colitis', *American Journal of Gastroenterology* 94 (1999): 427-433

4.Chey, W Y et al., 'Infliximab is an effective therapeutic agent for ulcerative colitis', *American Journal of Gastroenterology* 95 (2000): A2530

Chapter Eleven

1.Ekbom, A et al., 'Ulcerative Colitis and colorectal cancer: a population-based study', *New England Journal of Medicine* 323 (1990): 1228-1233

2.Farrell, R and Peppercorn, M *Lancet* January 2002: 331-340

ChapterTwelve
1.Bell, A M and Dozoi, R R, 'Elective surgical treatment for chronic
   ulcerative colitis', in *Inflammatory Bowel Disease*, editors Anagnostides, A A et al. (Chapman & Hall Medical, London 1991)
   p. 351

Chapter Fourteen
1.Thompson, W G et al., 'Functional bowel disorders and functional
   abdominal pain', *Gut* 45 (1999): 1143-1147
2.Sanders, D S et al., 'Association of adult coeliac disease with irritable bowel syndrome: a case-control study in patients fulfilling
   ROME II criteria referred to secondary care', *Lancet* 358
   (2001): 1504-1508

Index

Allergy.. 59-62
Alverine... 93
Antigliadin test... 95, 96
Arthritis.. 58
Azathioprine.. 39, 74
Bacteria............................... 22-27, 38, 48, 50-54, 63, 69-71, 75
Brooke, Professor Brian 33, 81-83, 89

Cancer 6, 33, 45, 49, 58-59
                                    77-79, 91, 92, 97-99, 101
Ciclosporin (cyclosporin).. 73, 74
Coeliac disease............................... 64, 89, 92, 94-96
Colpermin... 93
C-reactive protein (CRP).. 63
Crohn, Dr Burrell... 33
Cumming, Dr John... 90
Currie, Edwina.. 23

DALMs.. 78, 79
Dalziel, Dr Kennedy.. 33, 34
Diets:
– elemental 36, 62-65
– exclusion 64, 65
– formula... 64, 65, 85

Ekbom, Dr A... 77
EMA test... 95
ESR 63
Eye problems 37, 58, 68, 79

Fabricius, Dr P J.. 35
Faddy eaters.. 55
Farrell, Dr Richard.. 78
Farthing, Professor M G J... 36
Fartometer 90, 91

Fish oil.. 74
Fistulas 57, 85-87
Food intolerance.. 61

Gluten 64, 94-96

Ileostomy 81-86
Inflammatory Bowel Disease 6, 38, 39, 41-44,
48-51, 55, 61, 68, 81
Infliximab.. 39, 40, 49, 57, 59, 75
Irritable Bowel...6, 7, 17, 62, 89-96

Kock's continent ileostomy...................................... 82, 83

Lactulose 93
Laxatives.. 15, 16, 93

Mayo Clinic.. 83, 84, 86
Mebeverine 90, 93
Megacolon 86
Mercaptopurine.. 39, 74
Mesalazine 73-77
Methotrexate.. 39
Mormons.. 56
Mucosa.. 18, 22, 25, 41-47, 49,
51, 54, 55, 61-65, 67, 69-75

Nicotine.. 74-75, 78, 97-99, 102

Pan-proctocolectomy 81, 82
Peppercorn, Dr Mark.. 78
Pouchitis.. 74, 82, 83
Prednisolone 37, 73
Prince Albert.. 22
Probiotics.. 51, 74
Pyoderma gangrenosum.. 58

RCGPOCS.. 55, 56
ROME II 92, 93, 95, 96

Salmonella.. 22-24, 29, 42
Sanders, Dr David 95, 96
Shanahan, Professor Fergus 41-42, 45, 50-51
Shiga, Dr... 24
Smoking.. 55, 56, 68, 69, 78, 97-106
Stricturoplasty 86
Sugar... 9, 18, 28, 30, 36, 51, 53, 54, 62

Thalidomide 39, 49
TNF-α... 40, 49, 75
Typhoid Mary... 23

Valori, Dr R 95

Weaning.. 47, 54
Wolff, Professor B G 86
Workman, Dr E.. 63, 64